Learning More Biochemistry

100 NEW CASE-ORIENTED PROBLEMS

Learning More Biochemistry

100 NEW CASE-ORIENTED PROBLEMS

Richard F. Lodueña

Department of Biochemistry
The University of Texas Health Science Center
San Antonio, Texas

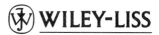

A JOHN WILEY & SONS, INC., PUBLICATION

NEW YORK • CHICHESTER • WEINHEIM • BRISBANE • SINGAPORE • TORONTO

Address All Inquiries to the Publisher
Wiley-Liss, Inc., 605 Third Avenue, New York, NY 10158-0012

Printed in the United States of America

While the authors, editors, and publisher believe that drug selection and dosage and the specifications and usage of equipment and devices, as set forth in this book, are in accord with current recommendations and practice at the time of publication, they accept no legal responsibility for any errors or omissions, and make no warranty, express or implied, with respect to material contained herein. In view of ongoing research, equipment modifications, changes in governmental regulations and the constant flow of information relating to drug therapy, drug reactions and the use of equipment and devices, the reader is urged to review and evaluate the information provided in the package insert or instructions for each drug, piece of equipment or device for, among other things, any changes in the instructions or indications of dosage or usage and for added warnings and precautions.

Library of Congress Cataloging-in-Publication Data

Ludueña, Richard F.
    Learning more biochemistry : 100 new case-oriented problems / Richard F. Ludueña.
        p.   cm.
    Includes index.
    ISBN 0-471-17054-2 (pbk. : alk. paper)
    1. Clinical biochemistry—Problems, exercises, etc.   I. Title.
    RB112.5.L83   1997
    612'.015'076—dc20   96-46129
                                                                          CIP

The text of this book is printed on acid-free paper.

10 9 8 7 6 5 4 3 2 1

To the best of fathers and the best of scientists:
Dr. Froilan P. Ludueña (1906–1982)

Contents

CONTENTS

Preface

Rereading the Introduction to *Learning Biochemistry* (1995), the previous set of 100 problems, shows me that I have relatively little introductory material to add to this new set of problems. Thus the previous Introduction is incorporated *in toto* in the following pages in which I set out how I decided to write this series of books and how the problems are to be worked and administered.

I do have a few comments, however, relevant to this book alone. The problems described here are based entirely on the very latest literature. All the problems were created beginning in August, 1995. One criticism of the previous version was that many of the problems could be solved fairly easily by recourse to a compendium, such as Scriver et al., *Metabolic Basis of Inherited Disease* (1989); by consulting this book, the students could obviate a more intense library search. The problems in this book, however, are based on literature so recent that there has not been time for the information to get into compendia. Where appropriate I have referred to Scriver et al., *The Metabolic and Molecular Bases of Inherited Disease* (1995); this marvelous work, however, does not contain the answers to the problems but does have some excellent background material and clinical descriptions.

I have continued to use the library projects in the course, giving the students a 4% bonus for the successful completion of their problem. The problems continue to be popular in the course. Most of the ones in this book were used for the first time in 1995. All of the students elected to do the projects (slightly above the constant figure of 98% in previous years). Of the 190 respondents to the evaluation, 60% rated their library project as "very educational," and 29% as "somewhat educational." Only 4% rated them negatively.

Many students consider the projects one of the most enjoyable parts of our Medical Biochemistry course. I intend to continue to create more projects as new advances are made in our understanding of the molecular basis of disease.

ACKNOWLEDGMENTS

I am indebted to many people for their help with this book. My teaching colleagues in our Medical Biochemistry course, Drs. Martin Adamo, Jeff Hansen, John Lee, Fredrik Leeb-Lundberg, Bettie Sue Masters, Barry Nall, and Merle Olson, deserve many thanks for their assistance and their support. I would particularly like to thank my wife Linda Lueña for suggesting one of the problems and Drs. Roger Kornberg and Jon Nishimura for their assistance with certain problems. I would also like to acknowledge my editors at Wiley-Liss, Drs. William Curtis and Stephanie Diment, for their support and wise suggestions.

Finally, I would like to thank the 20 classes of medical students whom I have been privileged to teach, particularly the classes of 1999 and 2000, who have been the guinea pigs for the problems in this book.

Introduction for the Professor

Genesis

I have had the pleasure and privilege of teaching medical students for the last 17 years. Although I enjoy lecturing very much, I recognize that there are limitations to the lecture system. In many ways it is a passive system of learning in which the professor expounds and the student memorizes. The syllabus and the text are in essence aids to memory. The examinations are in large part assays to measure the extent of memorization that has occurred. In this system the students take little responsibility for their own learning. Their questions are often driven by the desire to delineate with the highest possible exactitude the precise boundary between what is and what is not required to be committed to memory. In the scramble for grades, the beauty of biochemistry is easy to miss. Even if that beauty animates the lecturer, there may not be enough time to have it illuminate a great deal of the course content. Often, even in medical biochemistry, there is little time to expand on clinical applications of the corpus of information. This is unfortunate because, after all, the students are in medical school to learn how to treat patients; they want to see how biochemistry relates to real patients. Often, students resent what they perceive as a lack of "relevance." That is not to say that a medical biochemistry course has no clinical relevance. There is usually enough time to tell students about the biochemical basis of diabetes, hemophilia, and a few other diseases. There are, of course, a whole host of other clinically relevant topics that could be discussed were there time enough.

The size of the typical medical class makes it difficult to address some of these problems. When you lecture to 200 students, how can you relate to each one individually and talk to them about the aspects of biochemistry that interest them? For all of these reasons, there has recently been a movement to drop lectures in favor of small-group discussions and problem-based learning. Although these are excellent formats for learning, there are formidable logistical problems to overcome to restructure a curriculum in this fashion. I thought that it would be good to have a vehicle that could add a dimension of problem-based learning to a lecture-centered course or which could be used in small-group discussions in a nontraditional curriculum. I conceived of this venture as one that would add flexibility to the curriculum.

I created these library projects about three years ago. I made up about 230 problems, from which I have chosen 100 for this book. I wanted to oblige the students to use the library as a resource where information could be found. Naturally, I had to choose problems whose answers could not be deduced from the rest of the course material: namely, the textbook, the syllabus, or the lectures. For this reason you will not see any problems about diseases such as diabetes or classic hemophilia, whose etiology is discussed in most biochemistry textbooks. Our textbook is Devlin's *Textbook of Biochemistry with Clinical Correlations*, 3rd edition. As its name implies, this is a textbook with numerous clinical correlations; it discusses the biochemical bases of quite a few diseases. For the problems in this book, therefore, I have had to find other diseases, not discussed in Devlin's book. In a sense, this book is constructed around that text and is complementary to it. However, this book could be used just as easily to accompany any other biochemistry textbook.

I have assigned each problem to a pair of students at the beginning of the course and given them the rest of the semester to come up with the answer. Successful completion of the problem is worth 4 percentage points, added to the average of their scores on the three formal examinations. The problems are voluntary. Each year 98% of the students have chosen to do the problems. They have been very well received, with 58% of the students rating them as "very educational" and 31% as "somewhat educational." Fewer than 4% of the students rated them negatively. There have even been students who have asked to do extra problems for no extra credit.

The students are advised to show me the answers before turning them in. If they are incorrect or incomplete, I will not accept them. I will not tell them the answer, but I will point out how their answer contradicts the given facts. I ask them questions to get their thinking moving in a new direction. By this method, I get to interact one-on-one or one-on-two with about 80% of the students, thereby addressing the impersonal aspect of medical school referred to above. I might add that one of the greatest benefits that I have found in using these problems is that I get to know the majority of the students. This allows me to keep my finger on the pulse of the class and gives a very human face to the course. I can get a sense of each student's potential and personality.

Format

The format of this book is as follows. There are 100 numbered problems, covering many different areas of biochemistry. Each problem describes some kind of clinical situation, including the symptoms and some biochemical findings. These are followed by some short questions or problems, such as "What is the defective enzyme?" and "Write out the pathway in which this enzyme occurs" or "How do the symptoms arise?" or "How would you treat this patient?" At first glance some of the questions will seem very easy and some very hard. It is true that they are not of equal difficulty. However, three years of experience have shown me that my predictions as to which problems would be hard and which would be easy were way off target. Even the "easy" questions will require a trip to the library to answer. The process of researching the answer will be a serious learning experience for students. A few of the more difficult problems will require some elaborate reasoning by students. Occasionally, a hint is given in the form of a clue or even a reference to a paper to look up, but looking up this paper will not by itself solve the entire problem for students but rather help them narrow down what they are to look for or think about. The reasoning required by the questions is intended to exemplify and reinforce basic biochemical principles involving, for example, metabolic pathways, protein–ligand interactions, protein structure, and the genetic code. Students are expected to answer the questions briefly.

You may be worried that the "hard" questions are too hard. Rest assured that they are not. Do not think of these as test questions for which students have to carry the answers around in their heads; these are library projects. A trip to the library will fairly easily turn up the beginnings of each answer. The hardest parts of the questions are often the ones that you as professor would think are the easiest, because they require reasoning and relatively little information; for instance, if a disease involving a flavin-bound enzyme can be cured by increasing dietary flavin, the reason probably is that the defect involves the affinity of the enzyme for the flavin. This is an answer that is attainable by reasoning. Often, first-year students lack self-confidence in their ability to reason things out and turn instinctively to an authority, such as a book or other publication, to solve the problem. It is very good discipline for them to develop confidence in their own ability to think.

The book begins with a sample problem about familial amyloidosis, Finnish type. This is intended to show students what is expected of them. The sample problem is followed by the answer, including the reasoning that led to the answer. How much of the reasoning students will be required to show in their answers to these questions is up to the professor. I describe the reasoning to show students the basic strategy for answering these questions. There follow the 100 problems themselves, each group of problems being accompanied by their answers. You could photocopy a question and give it to students or use the question and its answer as the basis of a discussion. In many cases I have made the answers quite detailed, more so than is called for by the question. This will give you more latitude in judging student responses. Some students will answer the bare minimum; others will write volumes. Although students are not asked to name the disease, if the disease has a specific name, this is given in capitals at the end of the answer.

Where are the answers to be found? The students should go to the library and browse through texts or use computerized databases. Sometimes looking up the appropriate subject in the card catalog will lead them to the answers. Some of the problems are based on the very latest findings reported in the literature, so a computerized database will be necessary. Each problem is followed by a list of references that can be consulted for further information. If you have any suggestions or corrections about the problems, I would be very grateful if you would inform me.

Some of these problems are based on very rare diseases. You may worry, as I have, that students will object that you are asking them to waste their time on a disease that has been observed in only one or two patients. So far, no student has voiced this to me as an objection, but I have two answers ready. First, students will graduate as "doctors of medicine," not as "doctors of medicine specializing in common ailments." All diseases should be within the purview of a physician, not in the absurdly impractical sense that he should know all about them, but in the sense that he should be able to search, find, and understand information about them if they should happen to turn up. Second, and more important, these questions are not intended primarily to teach students about diseases but rather to teach them some biochemistry in an interesting and even exciting fashion and to show them that biochemistry is indeed relevant to medicine.

Administration

How the professor will use this book is entirely up to him or her. Here are some options to consider. At the beginning of the course, each student or group of students is assigned a certain number of problems. They could then turn in the problems with the answers at the end of the semester. They would be encouraged to work together, either in combinations assigned by the professor or in any fashion they desire. Their efforts will be graded and partial credit is encouraged; the scores they receive on these problems could count as a bonus, as an essential part of their grade, or as some combination of both. The problems could be discussed in conference sections, with the idea that the professor would not tell them the answers but rather, ask leading questions that could give the students an idea of where to look for the clues they need to get the answer. Students who turn in a sincere effort would get to see the answer to their questions. I would recommend not giving the answers to students who make no effort to find them out for themselves.

Of course, if enough students get to see the answers, what do you do for next year? This should not be a problem, since every week there appear in the literature new findings from which more problems such as these can be constructed. I intend to continue to do so.

In summary, this book is aimed at first-year medical students who are taking biochemistry and is intended to serve several purposes: to show students that biochemistry is indeed relevant to clinical medicine, to oblige students to take responsibility for their learning, and to teach students how to use the facilities of the library: general and specific reference books, the card catalog, computerized databases, and others. Finally, the problems are intended to be fun. If students have even half as much fun working on the problems as I did in creating them, this will have been a successful venture.

Introduction for the Student

This book contains 100 library projects in clinical biochemistry. Your professor will assign you one or more of these projects. Almost every one introduces a hypothetical patient or patients. A very brief account of the symptoms is followed by biochemical information in the form of an assay you may perform on a biopsy sample from your patient. Some questions also give you the sequence of a gene or a protein that may be altered in your patient. You are then asked various questions, such as to identify the defective enzyme, describe the metabolic pathway to which the enzyme belongs, and perhaps, to explain how the altered gene causes a defect in the enzyme or how the defective enzyme causes the symptoms. Keep in mind that in these problems, you are given the sequence of the "sense" strand of DNA. Unless otherwise indicated, all DNA sequences in this book are written in the 5'-to-3' direction.

The answers to these questions are not in your textbook or your syllabus. They will not be covered in class. To find the answers you will have to use the resources of your library. This will be excellent practice for later in medical school, when you will have to do research in the library in regard to specific patients. Look at the computerized databases in your library. The problem will give you some key words that may be useful for this search. You may also want to use the card catalog. For some problems your library may have a book that will give you the answer.

Keep in mind that looking up the problem in a book is only part of what you need to do to answer these questions. You will also have to think and use your judgment. Just because you find an answer in a book does not mean that the answer is correct. You may have found a book that is 30 years old and out of date. In general, go for the more recently published information. Remember that when you go to the library to learn more about your real patient's disease, the bottom line is to find the best information possible. If two sources contradict each other, you will have to use your judgment to decide which is more likely to be correct. You will have to reason out part of the answers to these questions using many of the basic biochemical principles you will be learning in your course. For example, when you were told that proline cannot be in an α-helix, you probably wondered what that nugget of wisdom had to do with a real patient. Some of these problems will demonstrate the connection as you use that piece of information to reason out how your patient's symptoms arise. Some questions will ask you to speculate. You will have to take your best guess, based on what you turned up in the library and what you have already reasoned out from basic principles. Do not be afraid to speculate; in the future, you will often have to do just that, deciding on the most likely course of action based on your experience and intelligence.

A sample question is provided here, based on familial amyloidosis, Finnish type. In this question you will see what you could look up and how you would apply basic biochemical principles to solving the problem. There is also some speculation required. These questions are intended to show you the relevance of biochemistry to clinical medicine, that many diseases have a biochemical foundation, and that understanding that foundation will help you understand the disease. Another aim of the questions is to make you familiar with the library and its resources. Still another is to help you develop confidence in your own thinking. Finally, based on my years on the admissions committee, I could predict that one thing that attracted you to medical school was the intellectual challenge; these problems are intended to provide some of that challenge and to be fun. I hope that you will enjoy them as much as I have.

Sample Question

Your patient began acquiring fibrous deposits in his cornea when he was 25. When he was in his 40s the muscles on his upper face started to become paralyzed. He is now 72. The skin on his face and his back hangs in loose folds. He suffers from a great deal of itching. You biopsy some fibrous deposits from his kidney and sequence the peptide component. Here is the sequence of the N-terminal region of the peptide:

Ala-Thr-Glu-Val-Pro-Val-Ser-Trp-Glu-Ser-Phe-Asn-Asn-Gly

You use your repertoire of molecular biological techniques to sequence your patient's gelsolin gene. Here is a portion of the sequence, compared to that for a normal person. Codon divisions are shown.

Your patient: CGT GCC ACC GAG GTA CCT GTG TCC TGG GAG AGC TTC AAC AAT GGC AAC TGC TTC
Normal person: CGT GCC ACC GAG GTA CCT GTG TCC TGG GAG AGC TTC AAC AAT GGC GAC TGC TTC

A full sequence analysis shows evidence for a repeating domain structure of 125 to 150 residues. There are six domains. The first domain has been crystallized and its three-dimensional structure obtained. From this the structures of the other domains can be deduced. One could therefore predict that the following structure would occur in the interior of the second domain of gelsolin:

a. Based on this information, how could the mutation in your patient lead to the fibrous deposits?

b. What is/are the functions of gelsolin?

c. Why does the disease not affect all of your patient's cells?

Answer

a. To understand the significance of the mutation in your patient, translate the nucleotide sequence into an amino acid sequence:

Your patient:
DNA: CGT GCC ACC GAG GTA CCT GTG TCC TGG GAG AGC TTC AAC AAT GGC AAC TGC TTC
RNA: CGU GCC ACC GAG GUA CCU GUG UCC UGG GAG AGC UUC AAC AAU GGC AAC UGC UUC
Protein: Arg Ala Thr Glu Val Pro Val Ser Trp Glu Ser Phe Asn Asn Gly Asn Cys Phe
Normal person:
DNA: CGT GCC ACC GAG GTA CCT GTG TCC TGG GAG AGC TTC AAC AAT GGC GAC TGC TTC
RNA: CGU GCC ACC GAG GUA CCU GUG UCC UGG GAG AGC UUC AAC AAU GGC GAC UGC UUC
Protein: Arg Ala Thr Glu Val Pro Val Ser Trp Glu Ser Phe Asn Asn Gly Asp Cys Phe

By looking up the sequence of gelsolin, you will identify this region as residues 172 to 189. Your patient has a mutation at position 187 in which an aspartate is changed to an asparagine (see figure). Why would such a seemingly minor change cause such a large outcome?

The X-ray structure of the first gelsolin domain shows that arginine 45 and aspartate 66 are oriented next to each other in the tertiary structure, and by deduction, arginine 169 and aspartate 187 should also be next to each other, in a position to form an ionic bond. Both arginine and aspartate are charged residues; the only way such residues could exist in the interior of a protein is if they are engaged in an ionic bond. The mutation of aspartate 187 to an asparagine, which is uncharged, leaves arginine 169 without a partner for an ionic bond. Hence arginine 169 has to move to the surface. This is bound to cause a change in conformation of the protein, which could by itself make it more susceptible to proteolytic degradation and aggregation. To understand this better, compare the sequence of the region of the gelsolin containing the mutation site with the N-terminal region of the protein that you have obtained from your patient's fibrils:

172 173 174 175 176 177 178 179 180 181 182 183 184 185 186 187
Gelsolin: Arg Ala Thr Glu Val Pro Val Ser Trp Glu Ser Phe Asn Asn Gly Asp
Peptide: Ala-Thr-Glu-Val-Pro-Val-Ser-Trp-Glu-Ser-Phe-Asn-Asn-Gly-

Clearly, the peptide was formed by proteolytic cleavage at arginine 172. This cleavage site should not be surprising; there are plenty of proteolytic enzymes in the blood (coagulation and complement factors) that cleave polypeptide chains after arginine residues. Why does normal gelsolin not get cleaved at arginine 172? Probably because the arginine is oriented in some way so as to make it less accessible to proteolytic enzymes. However, in your patient, the movement of arginine 169 to the surface makes it very likely that the position of the nearby arginine 172 will be altered; the change obviously makes it more susceptible to proteolytic cleavage. Once the proteolytic cleavage has occurred, the resulting fragment aggregates to form the amyloid deposits. Precisely what feature of the structure of this peptide predisposes to aggregation is not clear.

b. Gelsolin exists in two forms: One is cytoplasmic and one is found in the plasma. The cytoplasmic form plays major roles in actin polymerization. Actin is the major protein of microfilaments, which consist of two strands of actin molecules wound around each other in helical array. In many cells the microfilaments form a subcortical array adjacent to the plasma membrane and act as a gel to give some rigidity to the cell shape. Gelsolin can sever actin filaments. The first domain can intercalate between consecutive actin molecules in a single strand of the actin double helix. This leads to disassembly of the actin filament and to the dissolution of the gel, hence the name *gelsolin*. This would permit cell movement, shape changes, and secretion of vesicles that have to pass through this area. Gelsolin's actin filament-severing activity is induced by calcium and inhibited by the phosphoinositides phosphatidyl 4-monophosphate and phosphatidylinositol 4, 5-bisphosphate. Thus gelsolin plays a major regulatory role in cell movement, growth, and secretion. In addition, gelsolin, by virtue of binding to actin, can cap actin filaments and serve as a nucleation site for actin polymerization.

The plasma form of gelsolin is speculated to bind to and dissolve actin filaments that have been released into the plasma or the extracellular space as a result of tissue injury or cell death. This could be an important function since otherwise it is conceivable that these filaments could aggregate and precipitate.

c. If the explanation that you have derived above is true, why doesn't all your patient's gelsolin aggregate and cause trouble in all his cells? As mentioned above, there are two forms of gelsolin. They are identical except that the plasma form has an additional 25 amino acids. These two forms arise from two transcriptional initiation sites. A single cell can manufacture both sites. The mutation in your patient would therefore be in the cytoplasmic gelsolin as well as in the plasma gelsolin, which is the one that aggregates.

The reason the mutation does not have even more serious consequences is twofold. First, the mutation does not appear to compromise the function of gelsolin seriously. It has been shown that to exhibit the actin-severing activity, it is necessary to have only the first domain of gelsolin plus 20 residues from the second domain, up through arginine 169, and not including aspartate 187. This would imply that aspartate 187 is not necessary for this activity, nor is it necessary to have the arginine 169 in the interior of the protein. Also, one calcium and one phosphoinositide-binding site are located in the first domain, suggesting that a mutation in the second domain might not affect the regulatory behavior of gelsolin. Nucleation of actin filaments involves the last three domains. The second domain (which includes your patient's mutation) and the third domain are involved in filament binding. Perhaps the mutation does not compromise this function. In short, the mutation may not interfere significantly with the functions of gelsolin.

The second factor moderating the disease is this. Even if the mutation in your patient's gelsolin makes it more susceptible to proteolytic digestion, the altered gelsolin may not encounter, in his cells, proteolytic enzymes that will cleave at arginine 172 and generate the aggregating peptide. Thus only the plasma form is likely to come into contact with the appropriate proteolytic enzymes.

Your patient has FAMILIAL AMYLOIDOSIS, FINNISH TYPE.

REFERENCES

De la Chapelle, A., Tolvanen, R., Boysen, G., Santavy, J., Bleeker-Wagemakers, L., Maury, C.P., and Kere, J. Gelsolin-derived familial amyloidosis caused by asparagine or tyrosine substitution for aspartic acid at residue 187. *Nature Genet.* 2: 157, 1992.

Kwiatkowski, D. H., Mehl, R., and Yin, H. L. Genomic organization and biosynthesis of secreted and cytoplasmic forms of gelsolin. *J. Cell Biol.* 106: 375, 1988.

Kwiatkowski, D. J., Stossel, T. P., Orkin, S. H., Mole, J. E., Colten, H. R., and Yin, H. L. Plasma and cytoplasmic gelsolins are encoded by a single gene and contain a duplicated actin-binding domain. *Nature* 323: 455, 1986.

Maury, C. P. J., Alli, K., and Bauman, M. Finnish hereditary amyloidosis. Amino acid sequence homology between the amyloid fibril protein and human plasma gelsoline. *FEBS Lett.* 260: 85, 1990.

Mclaughlin, P. J., Gooch, J. T., Mannherz, H.-G., and Weeds, A. G. Structure of gelsolin segment 1-actin complex and the mechanism of filament severing. *Nature* 364: 685, 1993.

Meretoja, J. Familial systemic paramyloidosis with lattice dystrophy of the cornea, progressive cranial neuropathy, skin changes and various internal symptoms. A previously unrecognized heritable syndrome. *Ann. Clin. Res.* 1: 314, 1969.

Learning More Biochemistry

100 NEW CASE-ORIENTED PROBLEMS

CHAPTER 1

Lipid Metabolism

Problem 1

Your patient is a 42-year-old woman who weighs 396 pounds. When she was 20, she weighed 194 pounds. She is 5 feet, 9 inches tall. She has an alteration in the gene encoding her β₃-adrenergic receptor. The alteration is shown here:

Codon number:	62	63	64	65	66
Normal person:	ATC	GCC	TGG	ACT	CCG
Your patient:	ATC	GCC	CGG	ACT	CCG

Speculate on how the mutation could lead to or aggravate your patient's obesity.

Problem 2

You have a patient with adrenoleukodystrophy. You culture his fibroblasts and sequence a segment of DNA that is altered in your patient. The sequence of part of the DNA segment is shown here:

Codon number:	389	390	391
Your patient:	CTA	TGA	GAC
Normal individual:	CTA	CGA	GAC

You are able to purify the normal protein (X) coded for by this gene as well as the protein (X*) coded for by the altered gene. You do the following assay on proteins X and X*. You construct two peptides of the following sequence:

Peptide 1   Cys-Arg-Tyr-His-Leu-Lys-Pro-Leu-Gln-Ser-Lys-Leu
Peptide 2   Cys-Arg-Tyr-His-Leu-Lys-Pro-Leu-Gln-Ser-Glu-Leu

You measure the binding of the two peptides to proteins X and X* and obtain the following result:

	Amount of Peptide Bound (arbitrary units)	
	Peptide 1	Peptide 2
Protein X	100	5
Protein X*	5	5

In a second experiment you transfect the gene for protein X into some of your patient's fibroblasts and measure the rate of oxidation of radioactive lignoceric acid and obtain the following results:

Cell Source	Gene Transfected	Oxidation of Lignoceric Acid (nmol/h/mg)
Your patient	None	0.081
Your patient	Protein X	0.139
Normal person	None	0.191

3

In a final assay, you do immunohistochemistry of the cells with an antibody against the peptide Ser-Lys-Leu. You find that in the control cells the labeling is diffuse, whereas in those transfected with protein X the staining is concentrated in points, apparently in some small organelles.

    a. What is the problem with your patient's protein X?

    b. What is the basic problem in adrenoleukodystrophy?

    c. What is the function of protein X?

Problem 3

Your patient has Zellweger syndrome. You do a liver biopsy and homogenize the cells. You add 2-hydroxyphytanic acid to the homogenate and measure the production of 2-ketophytanic acid. You find that production of 2-ketophytanic acid in your patient's sample is 2% of the normal level. In the normal person H_2O_2 was produced in the reaction.

a. What is the defective enzyme and where is it located?

b. Write out the reaction that this enzyme catalyzes.

c. Write out the pathway in which this reaction occurs.

Answer 1

The mutation is analyzed as follows:

Codon number:	62	63	64	65	66
Normal person's DNA:	ATC	GCC	TGG	ACT	CCG
Normal person's RNA:	AUC	GCC	UGG	ACU	CCG
Normal person's protein:	Ilu	Ala	Trp	Thr	Pro
Your patient's DNA:	ATC	GCC	CGG	ACT	CCG
Your patient's RNA:	AUC	GCC	CGG	ACU	CCG
Your patient's protein:	Ilu	Ala	Arg	Thr	Pro

Your patient has an arginine at position 64 instead of a tryptophan. Position 64 is just at the beginning of the cytoplasmic loop between the first and second transmembrane domains in the β_3-adrenergic receptor. Replacement of a nonpolar by a charged residue at this place could easily cause one of two deleterious effects. First, it could move residue 64 out of the membrane and into the cytoplasm, thereby distorting the remaining cytoplasmic domain; this could interfere with the conformational change that is transmitted through the membrane when the catecholamine binds to the external domain of the β_3-adrenergic receptor. Second, it could alter the conformation of the cytoplasmic loop in such a way as to inhibit interaction with other proteins. Either way, one can imagine that this mutation could interfere with signal transduction.

The existence of the β_1 and β_2 subtypes of the β-adrenergic receptors has long been known. More recently, however, a third subtype, β_3, has been found. The β_3-adrenergic receptor is located in the membranes of adipose cells, particularly in brown adipose fat. It is also found in the intestine, skeletal muscle, and brain. The β_3 receptor has a lower affinity for catecholamines than do either the β_1- or β_2-adrenergic receptors. Presumably, it becomes activated when catecholamine levels are high, such as after a heavy meal or in response to cold. Once activated, the β_3-adrenergic receptor causes fat breakdown and also increases heat production. In mice, β_3 receptors are thought to be involved in stimulating synthesis of uncoupling protein, a protein involved in heat production in brown adipose tissue. There is speculation that the β_3 receptor in brown adipose tissue may mediate heat production in response to chronic cold exposure. If the receptor does not function well, one could imagine that less fat would be broken down than would happen in a normal person, and the result would be obesity.

REFERENCES

Arner, P. The β_3-adrenergic receptor—a cause and cure of obesity? *N. Engl. J. Med.* 333: 382, 1995.

Clément, K., Vaisse, C., St. J. Manning, B., Basdevant, A., Guy-Grand, B., Ruiz, J., Silver, K. D., Shuldiner, A. R., Froguel, P., and Strosberg, A. D. Genetic variation in the β_3-adrenergic receptor and an increased capacity to gain weight in patients with morbid obesity. *N. Engl. J. Med.* 333: 352, 1995.

Cummings, D. E., Brandon, E. P., Planas, J. V., Motamed, K., Idzerda, R. L., and McKnight, G. S. Genetically lean mice result from targeted disruption of the RIIβ subunit of protein kinase A. *Nature* 382: 623, 1996.

Granneman, J. G. Why do adipocytes make the β_3 adrenergic receptor? *Cell. Signal.* 7: 9, 1995.

Lands, A. M., Arnold, A., McAuliff, J. P., Luduena, F. P., and Brown, T. G. Differentiation of receptor systems activated by sympathomimetic amines. *Nature* 214: 597, 1967.

Liu, Y.-L., Toubro, S., Astrup, A., and Stock, M. J. Contribution of β_3-adrenoceptor activation to ephedrine-induced thermogenesis in humans. *Int. J. Obes.* 19: 678, 1995.

Lowell, B. B. Slimming with a leaner enzyme. *Nature* 382: 585, 1996.

Nisoli, E., Tonello, C., Landi, M., and Carruba, M. O. Functional studies of the first selective β_3-adrenergic receptor antagonist SR 59230A in rat brown adipocytes. *Mol. Pharmacol.* 49: 7, 1996.

Summers, R. J., Papaioannou, M., Harris, S., and Evans, B. A. Expression of β_3-adrenoceptor mRNA in rat brain. *Br. J. Pharmacol.* 116: 2547, 1995.

Answer 2

a. The alteration in the protein is as follows:

Codon number:	389	390	391
Your patient's DNA:	CTA	TGA	GAC
Your patient's RNA:	CUA	UGA	GAC
Protein X*:	Leu	STOP	
Protein X:	Leu	Arg	Asp
Normal individual's RNA:	CUA	CGA	GAC
Normal individual's DNA:	CTA	CGA	GAC

$$H_3C-(CH_2)_{22}-COOH$$

FIGURE A2-1. **Structure of lignoceric acid.**

Your patient has a mutation in which an arginine codon is replaced by a termination signal, leading to synthesis of a truncated and presumably nonfunctional protein.

b. Patients with adrenoleukodystrophy have badly functioning peroxisomes. A major function of peroxisomes is to oxidize very long chain fatty acids such as lignoceric acid (Fig. A2-1). Your patient clearly has difficulty with peroxisome function.

c. Protein X can restore peroxisome function. Therefore, it must be either a peroxisomal protein or a protein involved in targeting other proteins to the peroxisome. Proteins that are targeted to the peroxisome generally have C-termini ending in Ser-Lys-Leu. Protein X, but not protein X*, binds very well to a peptide ending in Ser-Lys-Leu. Also, when your patient's cells are stained with an antibody against Ser-Lys-Leu, transfection with protein X causes the stain to cluster in organelles that are presumably peroxisomes. It thus appears that the function of protein X is to recognize proteins with a peroxisomal signal sequence and to cause them to go to the peroxisomes.

REFERENCES

Dodt, G., Braverman, N., Wong, C., Moser, A., Moser, H. W., Watkins, P., Valle, D., and Gould, S. J. Mutations in the PTS1 receptor gene, *PXR1*, define complementation group 2 of the peroxisome biogenesis disorders. *Nat. Genet.* 9: 115, 1995.

Answer 3

a. Zellweger syndrome is a disease in which the peroxisomes are nonfunctional. Presumably therefore the missing enzyme activity must normally be located in the peroxisome. The enzyme converts 2-hydroxyphytanic acid to 2-ketophytanic acid. Since the reaction produces H_2O_2 as a by-product, it is likely to use O_2 as a substrate. Thus the missing enzyme is *2-hydroxyphytanic acid oxidase*.

b. 2-Hydroxyphytanic acid + O_2 → 2-ketophytanic acid + H_2O_2.

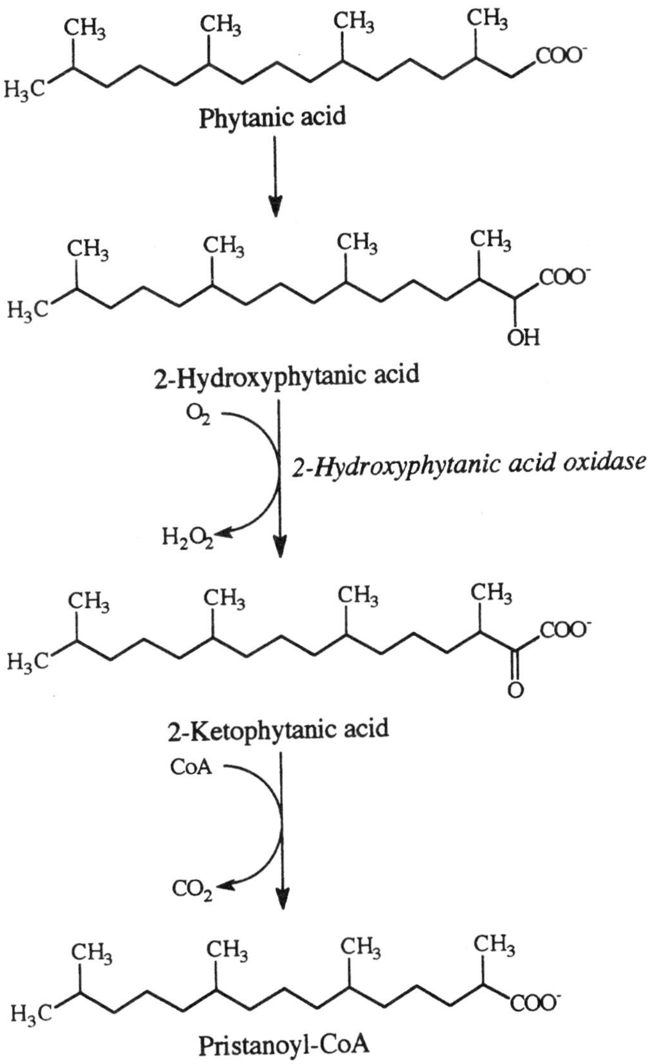

FIGURE A3-1. **Oxidation of phytanic acid.**

c. Phytanic acid → 2-hydroxyphytanic acid → 2-ketophytanic acid → pristanoyl-CoA.

REFERENCES

Wanders, R. J. A., van Roermund, C. W. T., Schor, D. S. M., ten Brink, H. J., and Jakobs, C. 2-Hydroxyphytanic acid oxidase activity in rat and human liver and its deficiency in the Zellweger syndrome. *Biochim. Biophys. Acta* 1227: 177, 1994.

Wanders, R. J., van Roermund, C. W. T., Schor, D. S. M., ten Brink, H. J., and Jakobs, C. Phytanic acid oxidation in man: Identification of a new enzyme catalyzing the formation of 2-ketophytanic acid from 2-hydroxyphytanic acid and its deficiency in the Zellweger syndrome. *J. Inherit. Metab. Dis.* 18: 201, 1995.

CHAPTER 2

Carbohydrate Metabolism

Problem 4

Your patient appeared normal for the first year of his life; then he lost his ability to walk and talk and even sit. His hearing is poor; he has trouble swallowing and is given to seizures. He also has an enlarged liver and spleen, coarse facial features, and a scaly skin. You have done a liver biopsy and prepared a cell extract. You add 2-hydroxy-5-nitrophenyl sulfate to this extract and measure the release of sulfate in the presence of NaCl. You find that sulfate release is much less than normal. You do the same experiment but replace sodium chloride with barium acetate. Again you find that sulfate release is much less than normal. To another sample of the extract, you add radioactive dihydroepiandrosterone sulfate and measure the release of radioactive dihydroepiandrosterone. You find that this is also greatly decreased in your patient's sample compared to what you would expect in a similar sample from a normal individual. Clearly, you have abnormalities in more than one enzyme. When you sequence the gene for one of these enzymes, you find that it is completely normal. You now purify the same enzyme from a normal individual and from your patient and subject them to tryptic digestion. You sequence the resulting peptides. One peptide from your patient (corresponding to residues 59–73) gave the sequence:

Phe-Thr-Asp-Phe-Tyr-Val-Pro-Val-Ser-Leu-Cys-Thr-Pro-Ser-Arg

You found a peptide with the same number of residues in the digest from the normal individual, which gave the sequence:

Phe-Thr-Asp-Phe-Tyr-Val-Pro-Val-Ser-Leu

The last five amino acids could not be identified.

You obtained some cells from your patient and from a normal individual and incubated them with [^{35}S]cysteine. You purified the above peptides and found that the peptide from your patient was labeled at the 11th residue, while the peptide from a normal individual was not labeled.

a. What is the defect in your patient and how might it cause the problem?

b. Describe the pathway that is defective in your patient.

Problem 5

Your patient has seizures and poor muscle tone. He has elevated levels of D-2-hydroxyglutaric acid in his blood, urine, and cerebrospinal fluid. You prepared mitochondria from a biopsy sample of your patient, added D-2-hydroxyglutaric acid and 2-(p-iodophenyl)-3-(p-nitrophenyl)-5-phenyltetrazolium chloride, a reagent able to accept electrons from $FADH_2$. You measure the change of color as the dye receives electrons; you observe that much less color change happens in your patient's mitochondria than in those of a normal individual.

a. What is the likely defective enzyme?

b. Describe the pathway in which this enzyme is likely to occur.

Answer 4

a. You have assayed three different enzymes. Arylsulfatase A and B both release sulfate from 2-hydroxy-5-nitrophenyl sulfate; arylsulfatase A is inhibited by barium ion and arylsulfatase B by chloride ion. You have low activity with each condition, thus both enzymes are defective. Steroid sulfatase releases sulfate from dihydroepiandrosterone sulfate; this enzyme is also defective. However, when you look at the gene for one of these enzymes you find that it is perfectly normal. The defect, therefore, is likely to be in a post-translational modification of a protein. The arylsulfatase A has a cysteine at position 69 which is not modified in your patient, but is modified in a normal individual. The modified residue must interfere with sequencing of the peptide. The nature of the modification is not immediately apparent. However, it must entail removal of the sulfur of the cysteine, since the peptide loses its radioactivity. In fact, the cysteine is changed to 2-amino-3-oxopropionic acid.

This is likely to happen in a variety of sulfatases since your patient has a global problem as if he lacked a bunch of sulfatases. In fact, all the sulfatases appear to have this modification. The role of the modified residue is not clear but it may take part in the catalytic mechanism. Without the modification, the sulfatases are inactive. The retardation arises from the deficiency of arylsulfatase A, which metabolizes cerebroside sulfatase. The ichthyosis arises from inability to hydrolyze cholesteryl sulfate by arylsulfatase C and the coarsening of the features and the enlarged liver and spleen are from the mucopolysaccharidosis ensuing upon inability of the other sulfatases to act.

A summary of the various sulfatases is given in Table A4.

The reaction catalyzed by steroid sulfatase is shown in Figure A4-1.

b. The putative reaction by which cysteine is modified in these sulfatases is shown in Figure A4-2. As you can see, we still do not know the exact pathway or all the reactants.

TABLE A4 Sulfatases and Their Natural Substrates

Enzyme	Substrates
Arylsulfatase A	Galactosyl sulfatide
	Lactosyl sulfatide
	Cerebroside sulfate
Arylsulfatase B	UDP-N-acetylgalactosamine-4-sulfate
	Dermatan sulfate
	Chondroitin-4-sulfate
Arylsulfatase C	Dehydroepiandrosterone sulfate
	Pregnenolone sulfate
	Androstenediol-3-sulfate
	Estrone sulfate
	Cholesteryl sulfate
Iduronide-2-sulfate sulfatase	Dermatan sulfate
	Heparan sulfate
Heparan-N-sulfamidase	Heparan sulfate
N-acetylgalactosamine-6-sulfatase	Keratan sulfate
N-acetylglucosamine-6-sulfate sulfatase	Chondroitin-6-sulfate.

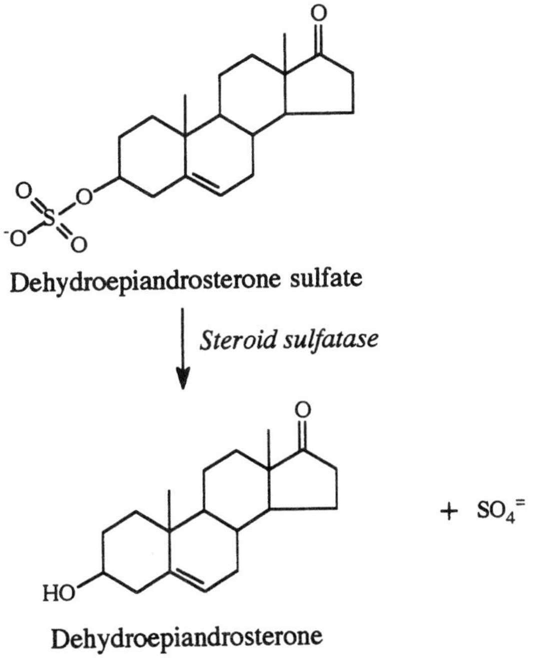

Dehydroepiandrosterone sulfate

Steroid sulfatase

Dehydroepiandrosterone

$+ \ SO_4^=$

FIGURE A4-1. **Steroid sulfatase reaction.**

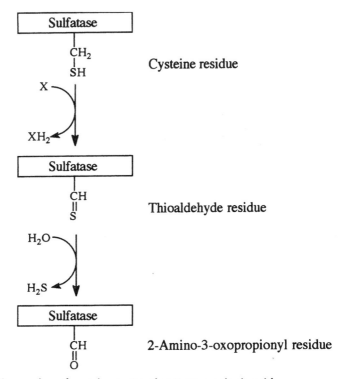

FIGURE A4-2. **Conversion of cysteine to 2-amino-3-oxopropionic acid.**

REFERENCES

Ballabio, A., and Shapiro, L. J. Steroid sulfatase deficiency and X-linked ichthyosis. C. R. Scriver, A. L. Beaudet, W. S. Sly, D. Valle, J. B. Stanbury, J. B. Wyngaarden, and D. S. Fredrickson (Eds.). *The Metabolic and Molecular Bases of Inherited Disease.* New York: McGraw-Hill, 1995, Vol. II, Chap. 96, p. 2999.

Baum, H., Dodgson, K. S., and Spencer, B. The assay of arylsulphatases A and B in human urine. *Clin. Chim. Acta* 4: 453, 1959.

Conary, J., Nauerth, A., Burns, G., Hasilik, A., and von Figura, K. Steroid sulfatase. Biosynthesis and processing in normal and mutant fibroblasts. *Eur. J. Biochem.* 158: 71, 1986.

Kolodny, E. H., and Fluharty, A. L. Metachromatic leukodystrophy and multiple sulfatase deficiency: Sulfatide lipidosis. C. R. Scriver, A. L. Beaudet, W. S. Sly, D. Valle, J. B. Stanbury, J. B. Wyngaarden, and D. S. Fredrickson (Eds.). *The Metabolic and Molecular Bases of Inherited Disease.* New York: McGraw-Hill, 1995, Vol. II, Chap. 88, p. 2693.

Rommerskirch, W., and Von Figura, K. Multiple sulfatase deficiency: catalytically

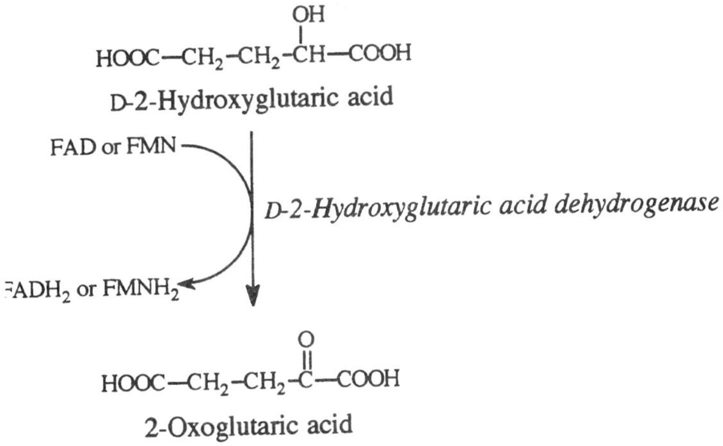

$$OH$$
$$HOOC-CH_2-CH_2-\overset{|}{C}H-COOH$$

D-2-Hydroxyglutaric acid

FAD or FMN

D-2-Hydroxyglutaric acid dehydrogenase

FADH₂ or FMNH₂

$$O$$
$$HOOC-CH_2-CH_2-\overset{\|}{C}-COOH$$

2-Oxoglutaric acid

FIGURE A5-1. **D-2-Hydroxyglutaric acid dehydrogenase reaction.**

inactive sulfatases are expressed from retrovirally introduced sulfatase cDNAs. *Proc. Natl. Acad. Sci. USA* 89: 2561, 1992.

Schmidt, B., Selmer, T., Ingendoh, A., and von Figura, K. A novel amino acid modification in sulfatases that is defective in multiple sulfatase deficiency. *Cell* 82: 271, 1995.

Answer 5

a. The defective enzyme is D-2-*hydroxyglutaric acid dehydrogenase*, located in the mitochondria. This is distinct from a similar enzyme called L-2-hydroxyglutaric acid dehydrogenase. The enzyme is a flavoprotein.

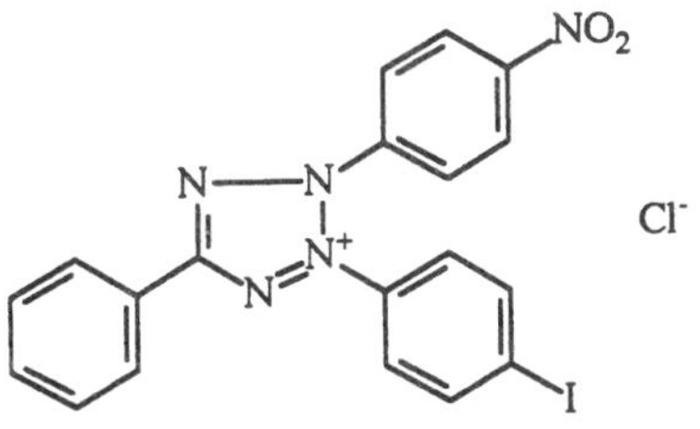

FIGURE A5-2. **Structure of 2-(*p*-iodophenyl)-3-(*p*-nitrophenyl)-5-phenyltetrazolium chloride.**

b. The enzyme probably transfers electrons from D-2-hydroxy-glutaric acid into the electron transport pathway, probably to coenzyme Q.

REFERENCES

Munujos, P., Coll-Cantí, J.,González-Sastre, F., and Gella, F. J. Assay of succinate dehydrogenase activity by a colorimetric-continuous method using iodonitro-tetrazolium chloride as electron acceptor. *Anal. Biochem.* 212: 506, 1993.

Nyhan, W. L., Shelton, D., Jakobs, C., Holmes, B., Bowe, C., Curry, C. J. R., Vance, C., Duran, M., and Sweetman, L. D-2-Hydroxyglutaric aciduria. *J. Child Neurol.* 10: 137, 1995.

Wanders, R. J. A., and Mooyer, P. D-2-Hydroxyglutaric acidaemia: Identification of a new enzyme, D-2-hydroxyglutarate dehydrogenase, localized in mito-chondria. *J. Inherit. Metab. Dis.* 18: 194, 1995.

Watanabe, H., Yamaguchi, S., Saiki, K., Shimizu, N., Fukao, T., Kondo, N., and Orii, T. Identification of the D-enantiomer of 2-hydroxyglutaric acid in glutaric aciduria type II. *Clin. Chim. Acta* 238: 115, 1995.

CHAPTER 3

Amino Acid Metabolism

Problem 6

Your patient exudes a strong smell of rotting fish. This is evident in his breath and sweat. This causes a great deal of stress for him; he has had to change jobs several times because of complaints from co-workers. He has elevated levels of trimethylamine in his urine. You are successfully treating him with metronidazole.

    a. What enzyme is likely to be defective in your patient?

    b. What foods would you counsel him to avoid? Why?

    c. What is the rationale for the metronidazole treatment?

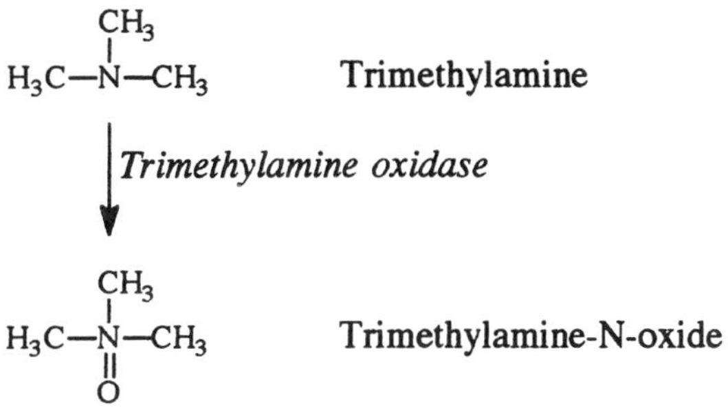

$$
\begin{array}{c}
CH_3 \\
| \\
H_3C-N-CH_3 \qquad \text{Trimethylamine}
\end{array}
$$

Trimethylamine oxidase

$$
\begin{array}{c}
CH_3 \\
| \\
H_3C-N-CH_3 \qquad \text{Trimethylamine-N-oxide} \\
\| \\
O
\end{array}
$$

FIGURE A6-1. **Trimethylamine oxidase reaction.**

Answer 6

a. Your patient is defective in *trimethylamine oxidase*, which converts the volatile and odorous trimethylamine to the non-volatile trimethylamine-N-oxide, which does not smell (Fig. A6-1).

b. Trimethylamine per se is not a common constituent of food, but our bacterial intestinal flora metabolize choline to trimethylamine. Hence, your patient should avoid choline-rich foods such as egg yolk, liver, kidney, legumes, and soy beans. Also, these bacteria reduce trimethylamine-N-oxide to trimethylamine, so your patient should avoid salt-water fish, which are rich in trimethylamine-N-oxide.

c. Metronidazole (Fig. A6-2) is an antibiotic specific for some anaerobic bacteria, such as *Bacteroides* and *Clostridium*. These bacteria are particularly effective in generating trimethylamine. Hence, antibiotic treatment can ameliorate this condition.

Your patient has FISH ODOR SYNDROME.

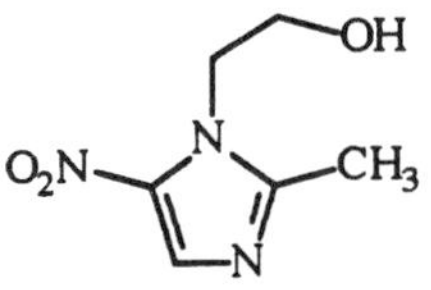

FIGURE A6-2. **Structure of metronidazole.**

ANSWER 6

REFERENCES

Treacy, E., Johnson, D., Pitt, J. J., and Danks, D. M. Trimethylaminuria, fish odour syndrome: A new method of detection and response to treatment with metronidazole. *J. Inherit. Metab. Dis.* 18: 306, 1995.

CHAPTER 4

Vitamins

Problem 7

In 1860, Robert Burke, John Wills, Charles Gray, John King, and several companions set out from Melbourne, Australia, heading for the Gulf of Carpentaria, in an attempt to be the first to cross Australia from south to north. When they reached Cooper's Creek, the four men left their companions to wait for them while they continued their trek alone. They were successful in reaching the north coast of Australia, but because of heavy rains they were delayed and ran out of supplies. On their return journey, they began to eat some fresh-water mussels (*Velesunio ambiguus*) and in a few weeks became sick. Gray soon died. In his journal Wills noted:

> *Our legs almost paralyzed so that each of us found it a most trying task only to walk a few yards. Such a leg bound feeling I never before experienced and hope I never shall again. The exertion required to get up a slight piece of rising ground, even without any load, induces an indescribable sensation of pain and helplessness, and the general lassitude makes one unfit for anything.*

When they reached their camp at Cooper's Creek, they found that their companions had given up on them and departed. They had, however, left behind a supply of oatmeal and sugar. Adding these to their diet, they recovered almost completely. As they rested at Cooper's Creek, waiting for a rescue expedition, their oatmeal began to run out and they began to subsist on flour made from the sporocarps of an indigenous fern called nardoo (*Marsilea drummondii*). This is a popular food among the Australian aborigines. Burke, Wills, and King would grind up the sporocarps and cook them. Soon their symptoms returned. Wills wrote:

> *King out collecting nardoo. I still feel myself, if anything, weaker in the legs, I feel myself altogether too weak and exhausted; the cold plays the deuce with us from the small amount of clothing we have. Mr. Burke suffers greatly from the cold and is getting extremely weak. My pulse are at forty-eight, and very weak, and my legs and arms are nearly skin and bone.*

Soon Burke and Wills died, with a substantial supply of nardoo flour around them. Shortly thereafter, King was rescued by the aborigines who fed him with nardoo flour until he had partly recovered. The aborigines ate their nardoo flour raw after first soaking it in water. They also drank the water they soaked it in.

King never fully recovered; he developed a peripheral neuropathy that made it difficult for him to walk, although he was healthy otherwise.

a. Of what did Burke and Wills die?

b. What is the toxic substance in nardoo flour and how does it work?

c. Why are the aborigines able to subsist successfully on nardoo flour?

Problem 8

Your patient is a 20-year-old wheelchair-bound man who exhibits an absence of deep tendon reflexes. The lipoprotein profile of your patient is normal as is his absorption of dietary α-tocopherol (vitamin E). However, the VLDL (very low density lipoprotein) of your patient has significantly less α-tocopherol bound to it than you would expect in a normal individual. You sequence a portion of his DNA that codes for a certain protein. Part of the sequence is shown here, compared to that for a normal individual. (The sequence begins at the beginning of a codon:

Normal person: CAAATCACTCCATCCGTAGCCAAGAAGATTG
Your patient: CAAATCTCACTCCATCCGTAGCCAAGAAGATTG

   a. What is the nature of the mutation in your patient?

   b. What is the defective protein and what is its role?

   c. How does the defect lead to neural damage?

   d. How would you treat this patient to prevent further deterioration?

Problem 9

(This problem is dedicated to my friend and colleague Mary Carmen Roach, *née* Estes).

It is the year 1506 and you are the court physician for Alfonso I d'Este, the Duke of Ferrara. Pretend that you have modern knowledge and the capability to perform some simple enzyme assays using present technology. Alfonso has always been a healthy man, as have his brothers, but he is very worried about his beautiful young wife, Lucrezia Borgia. On the night of August 5, 1503, Lucrezia's father and brother, who were living in Rome at the time, went to dine in the vineyard of Cardinal da Corneto. It was a cool summer night, and both men sat outside for a long time, enjoying the night air. A few days later, both her brother and her father were sick. Her father became feverish and dehydrated and died on August 17, at the age of 73. Lucrezia's brother was ill for another week, but then he recovered. The marshes near Rome have not been drained since ancient times; Ferrara is surrounded by marshes. Popular lore has it that marsh air is unhealthy. Because of the location of Ferrara, Lucrezia is afraid that she may fall ill like her brother and father.

To see if Lucrezia is more likely to be susceptible to disease than Alfonso, you ask Alfonso's permission to draw his blood and Lucrezia's. To extend the comparison, you need some blood from close relatives. Unfortunately, Lucrezia has no close blood relatives in Ferrara. You ask Alfonso if you can draw blood from his brothers Giulio and Ferrante who are serving life terms in prison for attempting his assassination. Alfonso tells you to help yourself to as much of their blood as you want. From the blood, you purify the erythrocytes and do the following two assays and obtain the indicated results.

In the first assay, you lyse the erythrocytes and add NADPH and oxidized glutathione. To some samples you also add FAD. You measure spectrophotometrically the rate of disappearance of NADPH and obtain the following results:

| | △ NADPH (μmol/10^{12} RBC/min) | |
Patient	−FAD	+FAD
Lucrezia Borgia	220	225
Alfonso d'Este	150	222
Giulio d'Este	130	215
Ferrante d'Este	148	220

In the second assay, you lyse the erythrocytes and add pyridoxamine phosphate and measure the production of pyridoxal phosphate. You obtain the following results:

Patient	Pyridoxal Phosphate Produced (nmol/g Hb/h)
Lucrezia Borgia	20
Alfonso d'Este	9
Giulio d'Este	3
Ferrante d'Este	8

a. Which enzyme in the d'Este brothers is likely to be defective? Show the reaction catalyzed by this enzyme and the pathway of which this is a part.

b. How does this defect connect to Alfonso's health? How might his heritage influence this?

c. What is it in Lucrezia's heritage that accounts for her normal levels in the assays?

d. What dietary advice would you give Lucrezia? Her eating habits are very different from her husband's. She is a light eater, while he is a massive man given to large feasts. Be careful in your advice; people who displease the dukes of Ferrara often meet swift and painful ends!

Answer 7

a. Burke and Wills died of beriberi. This is caused by deficiency of thiamine.

b. The nardoo plant, a kind of fern, has a substantial amount of the enzyme thiaminase I, which cleaves thiamine and transfers the pyridimine moiety onto an acceptor, or co-substrate (Fig. A7-1). Thiaminase I is to be distinguished from the less common thiaminase II, which simply cleaves thiamine without a co-substrate. By cleaving thiamine, this enzyme in effect created a thiamine deficiency in the members of this expedition. Interestingly, certain mollusks also have thiaminase I activity so the mollusks were also probably toxic to the explorers. Less is known about mollusk thiaminase I. It is thought that the mollusk enzyme can transfer the pyrimidine moiety onto another thiamine molecule.

c. Thiaminase I from the nardoo plant requires some co-substrates such as proline, hydroxyproline, or adenine. When the aborigines soak the nardoo flour in water, they separate the thiaminase from its substrates, which reduces its activity. Even eating the flour and drinking the water at the same time will dilute the thiaminase and greatly weaken its activity.

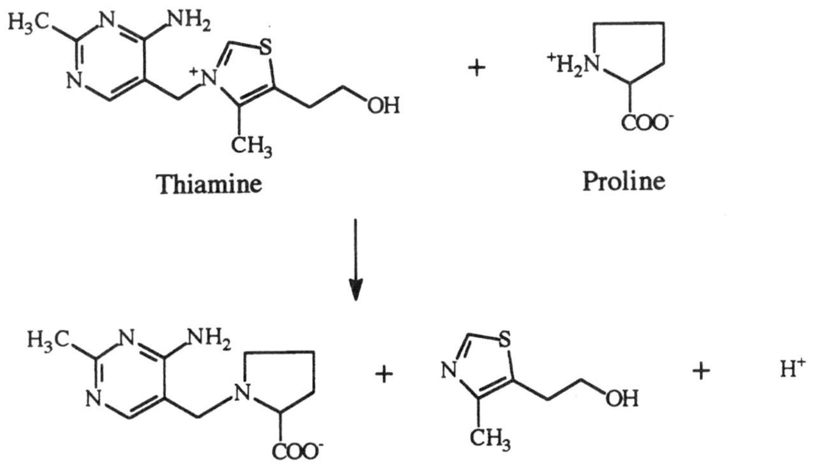

FIGURE A7-1. **Thiaminase I reaction using proline as a cosubstrate acceptor.**

REFERENCES

Earl, J. W., and McCleary, B. V. Mystery of the poisoned expedition. *Nature* 368: 683, 1994.

Evans, W. C. Thiaminases and their effects on animals. *Vitam. Horm.* 33: 467, 1975.

McCleary, B. V., and Chick, B. F. The purification and properties of a thiaminase I enzyme from nardoo (*Marsilea drummondii*). *Phytochemistry* 16: 207, 1977.

Ouzach, S. S., and Gorbach, Z. V. Characteristics of products developed after degradation of thiamin by mollusc thiaminase I. *Vopr. Med. Khim.* 35: 82, 1989.

Answer 8

a. First, look at the predicted sequences:

Normal person's DNA:	CAA ATC ACT CCA TCC GTA GCC AAG AAG ATT G
Normal person's RNA:	CAA AUC ACU CCA UCC GUA GCC AAG AAG AUU G
Normal person's protein:	Gln Ilu Thr Pro Ser Val Ala Lys Lys Ilu
Your patient's DNA:	CAA ATC TCA CTC CAT CCG TAG CCA AGA AGA TTG
Your patient's RNA:	CAA AUC UCA CUC CAU CCG UAG CCA AGA AGA UUG
Your patient's protein:	Gln Ilu Leu Leu His Pro STOP

Your patient has an insertion of two bases that causes a frameshift mutation that in turn leads to a STOP codon and premature termination of the protein.

b. The defective protein is α-tocopherol transfer protein. Its job is to transfer α-tocopherol (vitamin E) to VLDL (very low density lipoprotein). This is part of the recycling that allows vitamin E to be retained.

c. Vitamin E (Fig. A8-1). is an antioxidant that prevents damage to nerves.

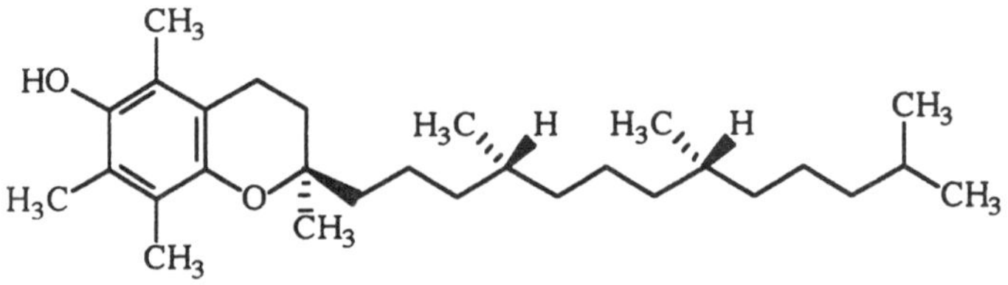

FIGURE A8-1. **Structure of Vitamin E.**

d. Further deterioration can be halted by giving your patient large doses of vitamin E.

Your patient has ATAXIA WITH ISOLATED VITAMIN E DEFICIENCY.

REFERENCES

Ouahchi, K., Arita, M., Kayden, H., Hentati, F., Ben Hamida, M., Sokol, R., Arai, H., Inoue, K., Mandel, J.-L., and Koenig, M. Ataxia with isolated vitamin E deficiency is caused by mutations in the α-tocopherol transfer protein. *Nat. Genet.* 9: 141, 1995.

Answer 9

a. The two enzymes being tested are glutathione reductase and pyridoxine phosphate oxidase. The first enzyme catalyzes the reaction (GSSG and GSH are the reduced and oxidized form of glutathione, respectively):

$$\text{GSSG} + \text{NADPH} + \text{H}^+ \xrightarrow{\text{FAD}} 2\,\text{GSH} + \text{NADP}^+$$

The second enzyme catalyzes the reaction:

$$\text{Pyridoxamine phosphate} + \text{O}_2 + \text{H}_2\text{O} \xrightarrow{\text{FMN}}$$
$$\text{Pyridoxal phosphate} + \text{H}_2\text{O}_2 + \text{NH}_3$$

The only factor that these enzymes have in common is that they use a flavin derivative as a coenzyme. Glutathione reductase uses FAD and pyridoxine phosphate oxidase uses FMN. If both activities are low, then it is likely that there is a deficiency of flavin, either in the dietary absorption of riboflavin or in its metabolism. The fact that glutathione reductase activity goes back to normal levels if FAD is added suggests that there is nothing wrong with the enzymes but rather with the FAD supply. The enzyme FAD pyrophosphorylase converts FMN to FAD. Since the FMN-requiring pyridoxamine phosphate oxidase activity is low, it is likely that the defect is in the FMN supply rather than the FAD pyrophosphorylase activity. Since

31

Alfonso is a big eater and quite overweight, it is likely that his diet is not a problem. The most likely defect, therefore, is in the enzyme *flavokinase*, which catalyzes the reaction shown here:

$$\text{Riboflavin} + \text{ATP} \rightarrow \text{FMN} + \text{ADP}$$

b. Lower levels of flavin mean lower activities of glutathione reductase in the erythrocytes. The malaria parasite lives inside erythrocytes. Low glutathione reductase activity means that the parasite is likely to be in too oxidizing an environment. This is thought to be deleterious for the integrity of the parasite's membranes. In addition, the malaria parasite appears to have high requirements for flavins. Thus, low flavin protects against malaria, a disease very prevalent in medieval Italy. Malaria is spread by mosquitoes that breed in marshes. In fact, the superstition about marsh air being bad was almost right. It's not the marsh air per se that's dangerous, however, but the mosquitoes that are in the air. Not surprisingly, "malaria" comes from the Italian phrase meaning "bad air." People in Ferrara have low flavokinase activities in their erythrocytes. This is simply an example of natural selection. Malaria has been a problem in Ferrara since the 1200s, about the time that the Este family left their mountain strongholds and took the reins of power in Ferrara. In the area of Rome, where Lucrezia's father and brother fell ill, malaria was a problem as far back as the second century BC, and, although improved by draining of the marshes by the Roman emperors, malaria returned after the empire disappeared.

Naturally, there is no way we can tell what kind of flavin levels Alfonso and Lucrezia had. One may question whether the 200 years that had elapsed since the Este took over Ferrara was sufficient time for Alfonso and his brothers to have developed immunity via a flavokinase mutation. After all, in the laboratory, one carries out selection among huge numbers of bacteria in a petri dish. A normal human generation is not likely to give such a large field for selection. In this connection, it is interesting to note that Alfonso's grandfather Niccoló III (1383–1441) had 3 wives, 800 mistresses, and 300 illegitimate children. He subsequently legitimized 22 of his bastard children. Three of these, including Alfonso's father, were rulers of Ferrara. Very likely, Niccoló only chose to legitimize the healthy ones who lived long enough to have him remember them. Certainly, only the healthy ones would have lived to become rulers. Thus, natural selection was probably given a chance to act. In fact, you might consider Niccoló and his children as a kind of human petri dish.

Alfonso and Ferrante are hypothesized to have had slightly higher enzyme activities than did Giulio. This is consistent with their parentage. Alfonso and Ferrante were legitimate and their mother was partly Spanish. In contrast, Giulio was illegitimate and his mother was probably Ferrarese. Hence, it is possible that Giulio may have had even more resistance to malaria than his brothers.

c. A quick glance at an encyclopedia will tell you that Lucrezia's parents were Pope Alexander VI and Vanozza de Cataneis. Her brother was the notorious Cesare Borgia. The low-flavin mutation is common in parts of Italy near marshes. Lucrezia's father, however, was not Italian, but Spanish. His family came from Jativa, a town in the hills of Aragon, near Valencia, and thus not likely to be a place troubled by malaria. Although Lucrezia's mother was Italian, if Vanozza was resistant to malaria,

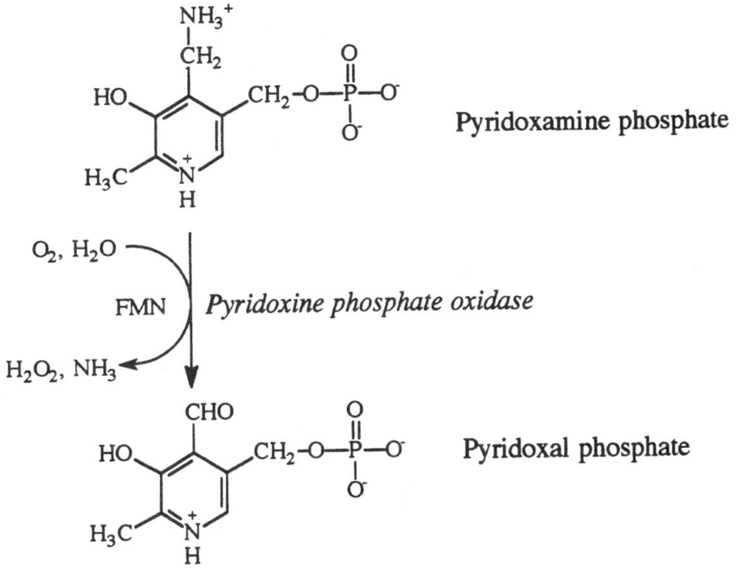

FIGURE A9-1. **Pyridoxine phosphate oxidase reaction.**

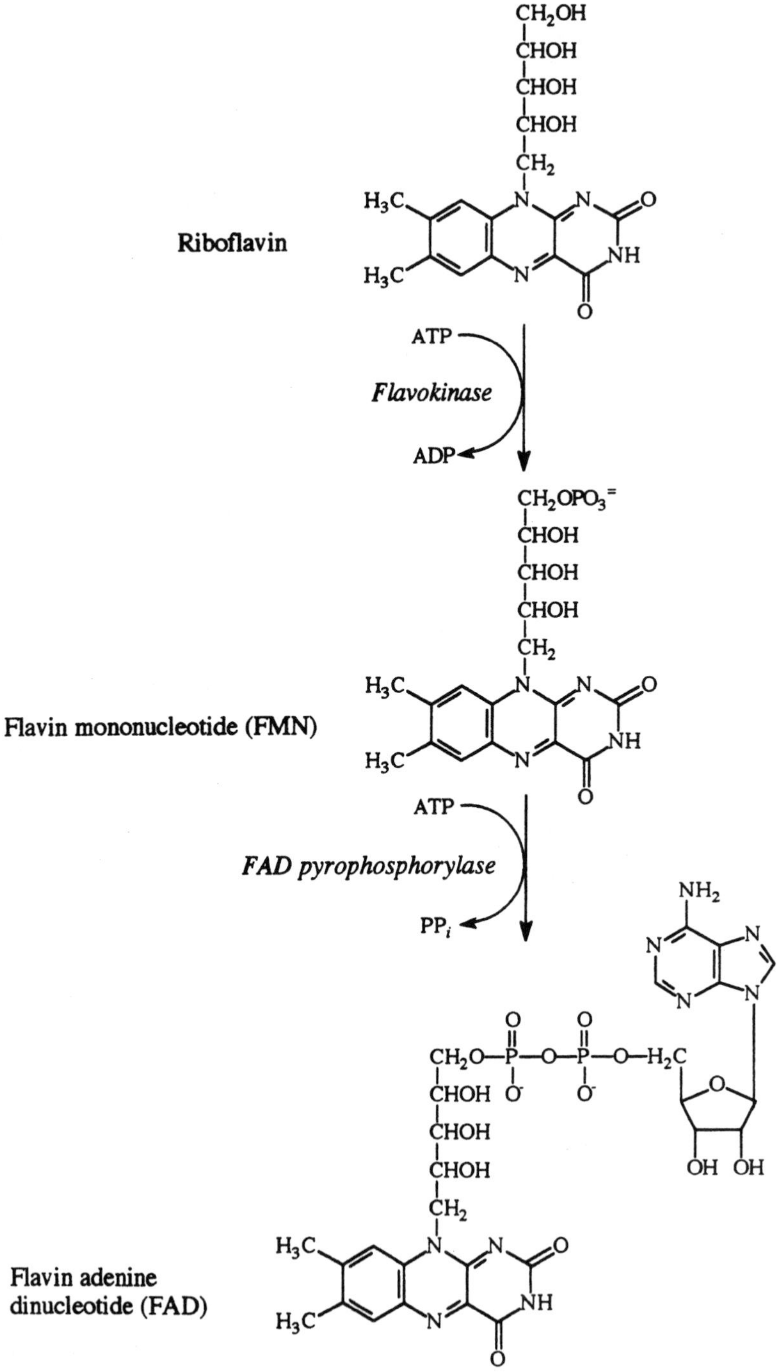

FIGURE A9-2. **Metabolism of riboflavin.**

she certainly did not pass her resistance on to her son Cesare and probably not to Lucrezia either. Thus, the Borgia family are likely to have been susceptible to malaria.

d. Studies in India have shown that children with riboflavin deficiency are more resistant to malaria. Thus, you would counsel Lucrezia to avoid high-protein foods, especially liver and kidneys, and to cut down on green vegetables. For her protein, she should drink milk, but preferably milk that has been exposed to sunlight for a while since ultraviolet light catalyzes the degradation of riboflavin.

REFERENCES

Anderson, B. B., Giuberti, M., Perrym G. M., Salsini, G., Casadio, I. and Vullo, C. Low red blood cell glutathione reductase and pyridoxine phosphate oxidase activities not related to dietary riboflavin: Selection by malaria. *Am. J. Clin. Nutr.* 57: 666, 1993.

Anderson, B. B., Scattoni, M., Perry, G. M., Galvan, P., Giuberti, M., Buonocore, G., and Vullo, C. Is the flavin-deficient red blood cell common in Maremma, Italy, an important defense against malaria in this area? *Am. J. Hum. Genet.* 55: 975, 1994.

Burman, E. *Italian Dynasties: The Great Families of Italy from the Renaissance to the Present Day.* Wellingborough, Northamptonshire, UK: Thorsons Publishing Group, 1989.

Clements, J. E., and Anderson, B. B. Pyridoxine (pyridoxamine) phosphate oxidase activity in the red cell. *Biochim. Biophys. Acta* 613: 401, 1980.

Clements, J. E., and Anderson, B. B. Glutathione reductase activity and pyridoxine (pyridoxamine) phosphate oxidase activity in the red cell. *Biochim. Biophys. Acta* 632: 159, 1980.

Cloulas, I. *The Borgias*, New York: Barnes and Noble, 1993.

Das, B. S., Das, D. B., Satpathy, R. N., Patnaik, J. K., and Bose, T. K. Riboflavin deficiency and severity of malaria. *Eur. J. Clin. Nutr.* 42: 277, 1988.

Dutta, P. Enhanced uptake and metabolism of riboflavin in erythrocytes infected with *Plasmodium falciparum J. Protozool.* 38: 479, 1991.

Dutta, P., Pinto, J., and Rivlin, R. Antimalarial effects of riboflavin deficiency. The *Lancet* 2: 1040, 1985.

Dutta, P., Gee, M., Rivlin, R. S., and Pinto, J. Riboflavin deficiency and glutathione metabolism in rats: Possible mechanisms underlying altered responses to hemolytic stimuli. *J. Nutr.* 118: 1149, 1988.

Fraccaro, P. La malaria e la storia dell'Italia antica. *Studi Etruschi* 2: 197, 1928.

CHAPTER 5

Minerals

Problem 10

Your patient has a type of cardiac arrhythmia called long QT syndrome. You have purified a protein from your patient and also cloned its cDNA. You express the normal protein in a *Xenopus* oocyte and measure the current across the cell membrane. You find that current develops only in the presence of added potassium. Your patient's gene has an alteration shown here:

Codon number:	625	626	627	628	629	630
Normal person:	GTG	GGC	TTC	GGC	AAC	GTC
Your patient:	GTG	GGC	TTC	AGC	AAC	GTC

a. What is the function of the mutated protein?

b. How might the mutation lead to the disease? Feel free to speculate.

Here are the sequences of portions of other proteins with similar functions to this one:

Mouse mSlo	Val	Gly	Tyr	Gly	Asp	Val
Drosophila Shaker	Val	Gly	Tyr	Gly	Asp	Met
Arabidopsis KAT1	Thr	Gly	Tyr	Gly	Asp	Phe
Drosophila Shaker mutant	Val	Gly	Tyr	Cys	Asp	Phe

The *Drosophila* Shaker mutant performed the same function as the wild-type Shaker, except that sodium could replace potassium.

Problem 11

Your patient has occasional episodes of tetany (severe muscle rigidity). Her serum calcium is considerably lower than normal as is her parathyroid hormone concentration. Infusion of EDTA (ethylenediamine tetraacetic acid) into your patient causes an increase in parathyroid hormone concentration in her serum. You clone and sequence a gene for a certain protein in your patient and find that it differs from that of a normal individual. Here is a portion of the sequence containing the alteration:

Codon number: 124 125 126 127 128 129 130 131 132
Normal person: TTG AAC CTT GAT GAG TTC TGC AAC TGC
Your patient: TTG AAC CTT GAT GCG TTC TGC AAC TGC

You take two batches of *Xenopus* oocytes and, in one batch, you express your patient's protein. In the other batch you express the normal protein. You then incubate the two batches of oocytes with different concentrations of calcium and measure the production by the oocytes of inositol 1,4,5-triphosphate (IP_3). Here are the results:

	Production of IP_3 by	
Ca^{2+} (mM)	Normal Protein	Your Patient's Protein
0.5	0.52	2.46
5.0	6.85	11.68

a. What is the mutation in your patient's protein?

b. What is the function of that protein?

c. Speculate on how the mutation leads to the hypocalcemia.

Problem 12

Your patient has liver failure and neurological problems. Biopsy shows large amounts of copper in the liver, while the blood has elevated copper concentrations. You prepare a protein from your patient and find that the protein has a histidine at position 1070 where that of a normal person would have a glutamine. Your patient's protein binds less ATP than does that of a normal person.

a. What is the role of this protein?

b. How does the alteration lead to the symptoms?

c. Why would you consider treating your patient with penicillamine?

Problem 13

Your patient has occasional episodes generally caused by stress, either physical or emotional, where he loses much of his muscular coordination. During these episodes, your patient has rippling movements of his muscles; sometimes these rippling movements occur without his having an attack. Your patient has an altered gene, a portion of whose sequence is shown here:

Codon number:	238	239	240
Normal person:	GTG	CGC	TTC
Your patient:	GTG	AGC	TTC

You express the patient's protein as well as the normal protein in two batches of *Xenopus* oocytes. You add radioactive potassium to the eggs and observe that the intracellular concentration of potassium in those eggs that have your patient's protein is much lower than the concentration in those eggs that have the normal protein.

a. What is the defective protein likely to be?

b. How might the mutation lead to the symptoms?

Problem 14

Your patient has just died. Autopsy showed very high concentrations of iron in his brain, liver, and pancreas. While still living he had diabetes and exhibited involuntary movements including facial grimaces as well as a lack of coordination. Concentrations of serum copper and ceruloplasmin were low. You analyze his ceruloplasmin gene and find that it is altered in an intron. You do the same analysis for the cerulopasmin gene of a normal person. Here are the partial sequences of both the gene and of a cDNA you make from the ceruloplasmin RNA (assume that it starts at the beginning of a codon):

Normal person's gene: CAATACAAGGTAGGA....TCTAATTAAGCACAGGGGAGTTTATAG
Normal person's cDNA: CAATACAAGCACAGGGGAGTTTATAG
Your patient's gene: CAATACAAGGTAGGA....TCTAATTAAACACAGGGGAGTTTATAG
Your patient's cDNA: CAATACAAGGGGAGTTTATAG

a. What is the nature of the mutation in your patient's ceruloplasmin gene?

b. How could the functions of ceruloplasmin explain your patient's symptoms?

Problem 15

Your patient has a muscle problem. When he attempts to exercise in the cold, his muscles tend to become rigid; at those times, he even has trouble swallowing. You have observed that he has an altered gene. When you clone the altered gene in a *Xenopus* oocyte and measure the ability of the membrane to permit sodium to pass through, you find that your patient's protein is somewhat less capable than that of a normal individual.

A portion of the sequence of the gene is shown here, compared with that of a normal person:

Normal person: TTA GGG GGG AAA GAC ATC TTT ATG ACG
Your patient: TTA GTG GGG AAA GAC ATC TTT ATG ACG

The protein is one with four transmembrane segments. The mutated amino acid is in an intracellular loop between the third and fourth transmembrane segments.

a. What is the role of the altered protein?

b. How might the altered protein lead to the cold sensitivity?

Answer 10

a. The protein that is altered in your patient is the major sub-unit of a potassium channel, known as the I_{Kr} channel. The gene that codes for it is called the "human *ether-a-go-go*-related gene" (HERG). It acquires its name because it is related to a gene called *ether-a-go-go* in the fruit fly *Drosophila*. When that gene is mutated and the flies are exposed to ether, they move their legs in a dancing motion; hence the name.

b. The mutation is analyzed as follows:

Codon number:	625	626	627	628	629	630
Normal person's DNA:	GTG	GGC	TTC	GGC	AAC	GTC
Normal person's RNA:	GUG	GGC	UUC	GGC	AAC	GUC
Normal person's protein:	Val	Gly	Phe	Gly	Asn	Val
Your patient's DNA:	GTG	GGC	TTC	AGC	AAC	GTC
Your patient's RNA:	GUG	GGC	UUC	AGC	AAC	GUC
Your patient's protein:	Val	Gly	Phe	Ser	Asn	Val

Your patient has a mutation at position 628 in which a serine replaces glycine. This glycine is highly conserved in evolution. Interestingly, in the *Drosophila* analog protein Shaker, the replacement of glycine with cysteine causes the protein to lose its specificity for potassium. It seems therefore that this glycine residue may play a role in determining the specificity of the channel in humans.

REFERENCES

Curran, M. E., Splawski, I., Timothy, K. W., Vincent, G. M., Green, E. D., and Keating, M. T. A molecular basis for cardiac arrhythmia: *HERG* mutations cause long QT syndrome. *Cell* 80: 795, 1995.

Heginbotham, L., Lu, Z., Abramson, T., and MacKinnon, R. Mutations in the K^+ channel signature sequence. *Biophys. J.* 66: 1061, 1994.

Sanguinetti, M. C., Jiang, C., Curran, M. E., and Keating, M. T. A mechanistic link between an inherited and an acquired cardiac arrhythmia: *HERG* encodes the I_{Kr} potassium channel. *Cell* 81: 299, 1995.

Answer 11

a. The mutation is identified as follows:

Codon number:	124	125	126	127	128	129	130	131	132
Normal person									
DNA:	TTG	AAC	CTT	GAT	GAG	TTC	TGC	AAC	TGC
RNA:	UUG	AAC	CUU	GAU	GAG	UUC	UGC	AAC	UGC
Protein:	Leu	Asn	Leu	Asp	Glu	Phe	Cys	Asn	Cys
Your patient									
DNA:	TTG	AAC	CTT	GAT	GCG	TTC	TGC	AAC	TGC
RNA:	UUG	AAC	CUU	GAU	GCG	UUC	UGC	AAC	UGC
Protein:	Leu	Asn	Leu	Asp	Ala	Phe	Cys	Asn	Cys

Your patient has an alanine at position 128 instead of a glutamic acid.

b. The fact that your patient responds to EDTA, a chelator of calcium, by increasing calcium concentration, suggests that the parathyroid hormone secretion is capable of being regulated and that the problem is not that there is a defect in the secretion of parathyroid hormone. The protein is likely to be a receptor that causes IP_3 to be made. It appears that the protein is very sensitive to calcium. Presumably it binds calcium with higher affinity than normal. The protein is the *calcium-sensing receptor*.

c. The mutation alters the hydrophobicity and perhaps the higher-order structure in the extracellular domain of the calcium-sensing receptor. The calcium-sensing receptor is expressed in the parathyroid, the thyroid, the kidney, and the brain. Its increased affinity for calcium may cause these tissues to think that the calcium concentration in the serum is higher than it is and, hence, they may take steps to lower it. This would account for the decreased parathyroid hormone concentration. A likely response by the thyroid would be to increase secretion of calcitonin, which would lower the calcium concentrations, leading to hypocalcemia.

Your patient has AUTOSOMAL DOMINANT HYPOCALCEMIA.

REFERENCES

Pollak, M. R., Brown, E. M., Estep, H. L., McLaine, P. N., Kifor, O., Park, J., Hebert, S. C., Seidman, C. E., and Seidman, J. G. Autosomal dominant hypocalcaemia caused by a Ca^{2+} -sensing receptor gene mutation. *Nat. Genet.* 8: 303, 1994.

Answer 12

a. Your patient has problems transporting copper, specifically in getting rid of it. We need copper, but only in small amounts, and our normal diet contains more copper than normal. The protein that is defective in your patient is one that transports copper.

b. The mutation is in the area of the protein that binds to ATP. The protein is a membrane protein that hydrolyzes ATP concomitantly with transporting copper ion. Inability to bind to ATP means the protein will not work and that copper will be deposited in tissues such as the liver and the brain leading to the observed symptoms.

c. Penicillamine (Fig. A12-1) is a chelator of copper. It will bind to some of the excess copper and lower the effective copper concentration.

Your patient has WILSON DISEASE.

REFERENCES

Thomas, G. R., Forbes, J. R., Roberts, E. A., Walshe, J. M., and Cox, D. W. The Wilson disease gene: Spectrum of mutations and their consequences. *Nat. Genet.* 9: 210, 1995.

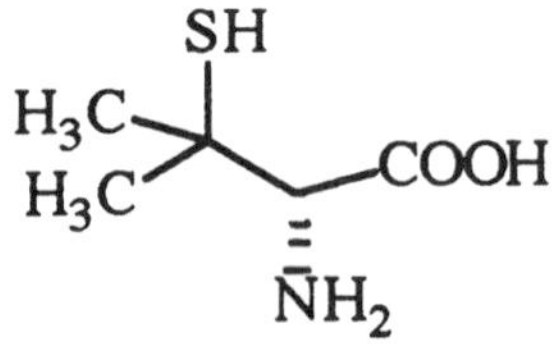

FIGURE A12-1. **Structure of penicillamine.**

Answer 13

a. The defective protein is a potassium channel, specifically, the product of the gene *KCNA1*.

b. First, identify the alteration in your patient's protein.

Codon number:	238	239	240
Normal person's DNA:	GTG	CGC	TTC
Normal person's RNA:	GUG	CGC	UUC
Normal person's protein:	Val	Arg	Phe
Your patient's DNA:	GTG	AGC	TTC
Your patient's RNA:	GUG	AGC	UUC
Your patient's protein:	Val	Ser	Phe

Your patient's protein has a serine substituted for an arginine. Changing a positively charged amino acid for a neutral one is likely to make great changes in the tertiary structure of any protein. In this particular protein, arg239 is in a transmembrane segment. An alteration in the structure of this segment may inhibit its function and lead to a closing of the channel. Since this protein is likely to be located in the cerebellum and peripheral nerves, if your patient has difficulty transporting potassium, it is easy to see why this could cause episodes of ataxia and spontaneous rippling movements in his muscles.

Your patient has EPISODIC ATAXIA/MYOKYMIA.

REFERENCE

Browne, D. L., Gancher, S. T., Nutt, J. G., Brunt, E. R. P., Smith, E. A., Kramer, P., and Litt, M. Episodic ataxia/myokymia syndrome is associated with point mutations in the human potassium channel gene, *KCNA1*. *Nat. Genet.* 8: 136, 1994.

Answer 14

a. First, you need to compare the two gene sequences. It appears that your patient has a G to A substitution (indicated with an asterisk). Second, you need to align the cDNA with the gene sequence to see exactly where the introns are:

Normal person's gene:	CAATACAAGGTAGGA....TCTAATTAAGCACAGGGGAGTTTATAG
Normal person's cDNA:	CAATACAAG CACAGGGGAGTTTATAG
Your patient's gene:	CAATACAAGGTAGGA....TCTAATTAAAČACAGGGGAGTTTATAG
Your patient's cDNA:	CAATACAAG GGGAGTTTATAG

As you can see, your patient has an altered cDNA sequence. The G→A substitution abolishes the AG splice site, so that splicing takes place at the next AG splice site, which happens to be in an exon. To see what effect that would have, you need to predict the amino acid sequences of your patient's ceruloplasmin:

Normal person's cDNA:	CAA	TAC	AAG	CAC	AGG	GGA	GTT	TAT	AG
Normal person's RNA:	CAA	UAC	AAG	CAC	AGG	GGA	GUU	UAU	AG
Normal person's protein:	Gln	Tyr	Lys	His	Arg	Gly	Val	Tyr	
Your patient's cDNA:	CAA	TAC	AAG	GGG	AGT	TTA	TAG		
Your patient's RNA:	CAA	UAC	AAG	GGG	AGU	UUA	UAG		
Your patient's protein:	Gln	Tyr	Lys	Gly	Ser	Leu	STOP		

The result of the G→A transition in the splice site is that you have introduced a termination codon into your patient's RNA, which means that he makes a truncated and presumably nonfunctional ceruloplasmin.

b. Ceruloplasmin is a copper transporting protein, but it also oxidizes ferrous iron to ferric iron, which makes the iron easier to transport. If the ceruloplasmin is defective, iron transport is inhibited and iron will deposit in tissues such as the brain (leading to neurological problems) and the pancreas (leading to diabetes).

Your patient has SYSTEMIC HEMOSIDEROSIS.

REFERENCE

Yoshida, K., Furihata, K., Takeda, S., Nakamura, A., Yamamoto, K., Morita, H., Hiyamuta. S., Ikeda, S., Shimizu. N., and Yanagisawa, N. A mutation in the ceruloplasmin gene is associated with systemic hemosiderosis in humans. *Nat. Genet.* 9: 267, 1995.

Answer 15

a. The altered protein is a sodium channel protein. If it does not work properly, the voltage across the membrane is not regulated correctly and the muscle becomes paralyzed.

b. The mutation is analyzed as follows:

Normal person's DNA:	TTA	GGG	GGG	AAA	GAC	ATC	TTT	ATG	ACG
Normal person's RNA:	UUA	GGG	GGG	AAA	GAC	AUC	UUU	AUG	ACG
Normal person's protein:	Leu	Gly	Gly	Lys	Asp	Ilu	Phe	Met	Thr
Your patient's DNA:	TTA	GTG	GGG	AAA	GAC	ATC	TTT	ATG	ACG
Your patient's RNA:	UUA	GUG	GGG	AAA	GAC	AUC	UUU	AUG	ACG
Your patient's protein:	Leu	Val	Gly	Lys	Asp	Ilu	Phe	Met	Thr

Your patient has a valine replacing a glycine in the cytoplasmic portion of the channel protein. In a normal person two glycines are followed by two charged amino acids, likely to be on the external surface of the protein. This is likely to be a rather flexible portion of the sequence. Flexibility may very well play a role in determining the function of this regulated protein. Replacing glycine with a much bulkier valine may decrease the flexibility of this portion of the protein. It is likely that, even if this change has no effect at normal temperatures, at lower temperatures, it may cause too much rigidity and thereby inactivate the protein and bring about the observed symptoms.

Your patient has PARAMYOTONIA CONGENITA.

REFERENCES

Hudson, A. J. Progressive neurological disorder and myotonia congenita associated with paramyotonia. *Brain* 86: 811, 1963.

McClatchey, A. I., Van den Bergh, P., Pericak-Vance, M. A., Raskind, W., Verellen, C., McKenna-Yasek, D., Rao, K., Haines, J. L., Bird, T., Brown, R. H., and Gusella, J. F. Temperature-sensitive mutations in the III–IV cytoplasmic loop region of the skeletal sodium channel gene in paramyotonia congenita. *Cell* 68: 769, 1992.

CHAPTER 6

Hormones

Problem 16

Your patient has cancer of the thyroid and the adrenals. You find that he has an altered gene. The product of this gene is a protein with three domains: an extracellular domain, a transmembrane domain, and an intracellular domain, the latter with tyrosine kinase activity. Your patient's mutation is in the extracellular domain. The partial sequences of the gene from your patient and from a normal person are shown here.

Codon number:	363	364	365	366
Normal person:	AAG	TGC	TTC	TGC
Your patient:	AAG	GGC	TTC	TGC

a. How might this mutation cause the symptoms?

b. More severe mutations in this gene often lead not to cancer but to a different disease where there is a lack of parasympathetic innervation of the lower intestinal tract, causing severe constipation, failure to thrive, and death. Speculate on how a different mutation in the same gene could lead to a very different disease.

Problem 17

Your patient is an apparent hermaphrodite, genetically a male with female external genitalia and with enlarged adrenals. Except for cholesterol, all steroid hormone levels are very low. You find that there is an altered gene in your patient, leading to an altered gene product, which we will call protein X. Part of the sequence of this gene is shown here, compared to that of the same protein from a normal individual:

Codon number:	191	192	193	194	195
Normal person:	AAG	CGC	CGA	GGC	TCC
Your patient:	AAG	CGC	CTA	GGC	TCC

Further analysis shows that cytochrome $P450_{scc}$ is normal in your patient.

You take three batches of COS-1 monkey kidney cells and transfect into all of the batches normal cytochrome $P450_{scc}$, adrenodoxin, and adrenodoxin reductase. Then, to one batch you transfect your patient's mutated gene and into the second batch the same gene from a normal individual. To the third batch, which is a control, you transfect only the carrier vector. Then to each batch you add either radioactive cholesterol or radioactive 20α-hydroxycholesterol (20α-OH) and measure the production of radioactive pregnenolone. You also prepare an antibody against protein X for a normal person and measure the amount in the two batches of cells. The results of these experiments are shown here:

Cells Transfected with	Pregenolone Production from		Protein X Level
	Cholesterol	20α-OH	
Control	20	158	0
Protein X (normal)	175	138	70
Protein X (mutated)	19	99	0

a. What protein is defective in your patient and what is the role of this protein?

b. How does the mutation lead to the defective protein?

Problem 18

Your patient is an infant with very low serum concentrations of glucocorticoids, aldosterone, and androgens. Injection of ACTH (adrenocorticotropic hormone) does not stimulate adrenal hormone production. You have identified a mutant gene in your patient. You transfect the normal gene into *Escherichia coli* and purify the gene product. The gene product is a protein (called protein X) with an interesting set of properties. First, using an antibody to it, you find that it localizes exclusively to nuclei and not to the cytoplasm. Second, it has homology in part of the sequence to the ligand-binding portion of various nuclear hormone receptors. Third, it has no domain homologous to the DNA-binding domain of the known nuclear hormone receptors.

You do an experiment in which you test the ability of the protein to bind both to the DNA segment that binds to retinoic acid receptors (segment 1) and to a DNA segment that does not bind to retinoic acid receptors (segment 2). You also see if it competes with a retinoic acid receptor (RAR) protein for binding to the DNA. Here are the results:

Protein Tested	DNA Segment Tested	Amount of Protein X Bound (arbitrary units)
Protein X	Segment 1	100
Protein X	Segment 2	0
Protein X + RAR	Segment 1	50
Protein X + RAR	Segment 2	0

What is the likely function of protein X?

Problem 19

Your patient has an unusual constellation of symptoms. He has premature development of pubic hairs and male genitalia (precocious puberty) and also has low calcium and high phosphate in his blood. A thyroid biopsy of cells kept at 37° C shows that addition of thyroid-stimulating hormone to these cells does not cause an increase in the release of thyroid hormone.

You find that he has an altered protein (called protein X). The protein has an alanine at position 366 where the normal protein has a serine. The protein is present in his testes but not in his parathyroid cells or his thyroid cells, although in a normal person, the protein would be present in all the tissues. You do the following experiments:

1. You cause both your patient's protein X and a normal protein X to be expressed in Sf9 cells; you then lyse the cells and add GTP labeled with radioactive phosphate at the γ position and measure the rate of hydrolysis of the GTP. In a separate experiment with the same type of cells, you measure the rate of synthesis of cAMP, but you don't add GTP to these cells. Here are the results:

Source of Protein X	GTP Hydrolysis	cAMP Production
Your patient	3.5 min^{-1}	80 pmol/mg/min
Normal person	0.18 min^{-1}	5 pmol/mg/min

2. You transfect the gene for protein X into TM3 cells and measure the production of cAMP at both 33° C and 37° C. You also measure the expression of the protein in these cells at both of these temperatures. Here are the results:

Source of Protein X	Temperature	Expression of Protein	cAMP Produced
Your patient	37° C	No	4
Your patient	33° C	Yes	16
Normal person	37° C	Yes	2
Normal person	33° C	Yes	2

3. You purify protein X both from your patient's cells and from a normal person and incubate it at 20° C either by itself or in the presence of either GTP or GDP. At different time points you remove an aliquot and measure its ability to bind to radioactive GTP-γS (an analog of GTP that hydrolyzes very slowly). What you are measuring is the rate at which the ability to bind to GTP-γS disappears. Here are the results:

Source of Protein	Nucleotide Added	Rate of Loss of Ability to Bind to GTP-γS
Your patient	None	0.34 min^{-1}
Your patient	GDP	0.087 min^{-1}
Your patient	GTP	0.023 min^{-1}
Normal person	None	0.013 min^{-1}
Normal person	GDP	0.001 min^{-1}
Normal person	GTP	0.001 min^{-1}

4. You measure the rate at which GDP bound to each protein is released. The results are the following:

Source of Protein	Rate of Release of Bound GDP
Your patient	14 min^{-1}
Normal person	0.18 min^{-1}

a. Why does your patient have precocious puberty? How does the mutation lead to this effect?

b. Why does your patient have resistance to thyroid-stimulating hormone?

c. Why is the protein present in your patient's testes but not in the thyroid or parathyroid?

Problem 20

Your patient has very low levels of calcium and of parathyroid hormone in his blood. Of his two brothers, one has the disease. Neither of his parents have the disease, but his paternal grandfather and his maternal grandfather are brothers. You find that your patient has a mutation in his gene for parathyroid hormone. Here is the structure of the parathyroid hormone gene in a normal individual:

Exon 1	Intron 1	Exon 2	Intron 2	Exon 3
85 bp	3019 bp	90 bp	103 bp	612 bp

Exon 1 is untranslated. Exon 2 codes for the signal peptide and part of the prosequence. Exon 3 codes for the rest of the prosequence and for the hormone itself.

The sequence of the exon 2–intron 2 boundary for your patient and for a normal person are shown (exons are capitalized, introns are not):

Normal person: CTGTTAAgtaagtac
Your patient: CTGTTAActaagtac

The 3' end of exon 1 in a normal person is shown here:

CATTGTATG

The 5' end of exon 3 in a normal person is shown here:

GAAGAGATC

When you examine the expression of your patient's PTH gene, you find that a normal person's cDNA is 787 bp, while your patient's is 697 bp.

You find the following sequence in your patient's cDNA:

CATTGTATGGAAGAGATC

a. Describe how the observed mutation leads to the disease.
b. What is the significance of his parents being first cousins?

Answer 16

a. The mutation is analyzed as follows:

Codon number:	363	364	365	366
Normal person's DNA:	AAG	TGC	TTC	TGC
Normal person's RNA:	AAG	UGC	UUC	UGC
Normal person's protein:	Lys	Cys	Phe	Cys
Your patient's DNA:	AAG	GGC	TTC	TGC
Your patient's RNA:	AAG	GGC	UUC	UGC
Your patient's protein:	Lys	Gly	Phe	Cys

Your patient has a glycine instead of a cysteine at position 364. This is the cysteine-rich domain of the protein. The protein is called *receptor tyrosine kinase (RET)*. It is not clear what the normal ligand of this receptor is. Presumably whatever it is leads to activation of the tyrosine kinase activity, which in turn activates other enzymes and may cause cell division as part of the normal developmental process. Conceivably, altering the cysteine-rich domain may affect ligand binding. It is possible that the mutation turns the protein on constitutively, in other words, that it may become unregulated and continually send signals for the cell to divide. In individuals who for some reason may lack other controls in those cells, it may lead to cancer.

b. Proteins of this type play important roles in development. Possibly mutations that wipe out *RET* activity may cause certain cells to lose the ability to respond to certain signals that trigger their growth during embryonic development. If this is the case, then one can imagine that the parasympathetic nerves to the lower intestinal tract may never develop. The *RET* gene is widespread in the body. It is interesting to speculate why the effects of *RET* mutations are relatively localized. Probably there are redundancies in the systems that control growth and development. Certain cells may have a backup so that if the *RET* gene works inappropriately, the deleterious effect may be ameliorated; hence, the effects would be limited to cells that lacked the backup systems.

Your patient has MULTIPLE ENDOCRINE NEOPLASIA TYPE 2A.

REFERENCES

Mulligan, L. M., Kwok, J. B. J., Healey, C. S., Elsdon, M. J., Eng, C., Gardner, E., Love, D. R., Mole, S. E., Moore, J. K., Papi, L., Ponder, M. A., Telenius, H., Tunnacliffe, A., and Ponder, B. A. J. Germ-line mutations of the *RET* proto-oncogene in multiple endocrine neoplasia type 2A. *Nature* 363: 458, 1993.

Van Heyningen, V. One gene—four syndromes. *Nature* 367: 319, 1994.

Answer 17

a. The enzyme that converts cholesterol to pregnenolone is cytochrome $P450_{scc}$. It does this in a reaction whose first step is conversion of cholesterol to 20α-hydroxycholesterol. However, we are told that this enzyme is normal in your patient. Nevertheless, the control batch of cells, which have cytochrome $P450_{scc}$, are unable to metabolize cholesterol. Therefore, the defective enzyme must be something else. The likely candidate is the protein that transports cholesterol across the inner mitochondrial membrane, which is *steroidogenic acute regulatory* (StAR) *protein*. Without this protein, cholesterol will not cross the mitochondrial membrane, but 20α-hydroxycholesterol can diffuse fairly well. This is why pregnenolone can be produced in all the cells even in the absence of normal StAR, if 20α-hydroxycholesterol is the substrate.

b. The mutation is analyzed as follows:

Codon number:	191	192	193	194	195
Normal person's DNA:	AAG	CGC	CGA	GGC	TCC
Normal person's RNA:	AAG	CGC	CGA	GGC	UCC
Normal person's protein:	Lys	Arg	Arg	Gly	Ser
Your patient's DNA:	AAG	CGC	CTA	GGC	TCC
Your patient's RNA:	AAG	CGC	CUA	GGC	UCC
Your patient's protein:	Lys	Arg	Leu	Gly	Ser

Your patient has a leucine at position 193 instead of an arginine. This is likely to have large conformational changes in the protein since a charged amino acid is replaced by a hydrophobic one. It is possible that the arginine is on the exterior and that the leucine moves toward the interior; alternatively, the arginine could have been participating in an electrostatic bond in the interior, a bond that would no longer be possible. Either way, profound conformational consequences are a likely result of the mutation. The fact that the antibody does not bind to your patient's protein when it is expressed in the COS-1 cells, however, suggests something more. A missense mutation should not completely abolish antibody binding. Probably, the mutation, perhaps by a drastic change in the conformation, inhibits the processing of the protein in such a way that it is either never properly transported into the mitochondria and hence may become degraded or else it is degraded after transport into the mitochondria.

Your patient has CONGENITAL LIPOID ADRENAL HYPER-PLASIA.

REFERENCES

Lin, D., Sugawara, T., Strauss, J. F., Clark, B. J., Stocco, D. M., Saenger, P., Rogol, A., and Miller, W. L. Role of steroidogenic acute regulatory protein in adrenal and gonadal steroidogenesis. *Science* 267: 1828, 1995.

Waterman, M. R. A rising StAR: an essential role in cholesterol transport. *Science* 267: 1780, 1995.

Answer 18

Protein X localizes to the nucleus and has a homology to other nuclear hormone receptors at their ligand-binding site. Protein X also binds to DNA and specifically to a site that binds to another nuclear hormone receptor (retinoic acid receptor). Thus, protein X is likely to be a nuclear hormone receptor with an unusual DNA-binding domain. Binding of protein X to DNA is inhibited by binding of a retinoic acid receptor, suggesting that protein X is involved in the retinoic-acid-induced regulation of development. Presumably, protein X inhibits the binding of retinoic acid receptor to DNA and hence inhibits transcription induced by receptor binding. Protein X must act at a critical developmental stage in which retinoic acid is involved in causing the adrenal gland to develop. Mutations in protein X could thus lead to inappropriate development of the adrenal.

Your patient has X-LINKED ADRENAL HYPOPLASIA CONGENITA.

REFERENCES

Zanaria, E., Muscatelli, F., Bardoni, B., Strom, T. M., Guioli, S., Guo, W., Lalli, E., Moser, C., Walker, A. P., McCabe, E. R. B., Meitinger, T., Monaco, A. P., Sassone-Corsi, P., and Camerino G. An unusual member of the nuclear hormone receptor superfamily responsible for X-linked adrenal hypolasia congenita. *Nature* 372: 635, 1994.

Answer 19

a. The defective protein is likely to be a component of a system that responds to both luteinizing hormone and to thyroid-stimulating hormone. The fact that it binds to guanine nucleotides suggests that it is a G protein. In fact it is the G_α protein. Clearly, the altered protein hydrolyzes GTP very rapidly and thereby causes cAMP to be made rapidly, even in the absence of added signal. In other words, the Leydig cells of the testis are turned on and making testosterone even in a preadolescent boy. In a normal boy, the increase in testosterone synthesis is dependent on the increase in luteinizing hormone release that accompanies puberty. Hence, your patient has precocious puberty.

b. Thyroid-stimulating hormone works by activating an adenyl cyclase via a G_α protein. Obviously, your patient lacks the G_α protein in his thyroid. Hence, the binding of thyroid-stimulating hormone to the receptor will have no effect.

c. The testes are cooler than the rest of the body. The mutated G_α protein is temperature sensitive. In fact, the reason why it hydrolyzes GTP so well is that it quickly loses the bound GDP, thereby allowing GTP to replace it. Guanine nucleotides clearly play a role in stabilizing the protein. Your patient's protein is less stable. At 37° C, the mutated G_α protein is rapidly degraded. In the cooler testes, however, the protein is not degraded but continues to function, even though its functioning is deleterious.

Your patient has TESTOTOXICOSIS WITH PSEUDOHYPO-PARATHYROIDISM TYPE 1a.

REFERENCES

Iiri, T., Herzmark, P., Nakamoto, J. M., Van Dop, C., and Bourne, H. R. Rapid GDP release from $G_{s\alpha}$ in patients with gain and loss of endocrine function. *Nature* 371: 164, 1994.

Nakamoto, J. M., Jones, E. A., Zimmerman, D., Scott, M. L., Donlan, M. A., and Van Dop, C. A missense mutation in the $G_s\alpha$ gene is associated with pseudo-hypothyroidism type I-A (PHP0IA) and gonadotropin-independent precocious puberty (GIPP). *Clin. Res.* 41: 40A, 1993.

Noel, J. P., Hamm, H. E., and Sigler, P. B. The 2.2 Å crystal structure of transducin-α complexed with GTPγS. *Nature* 366: 654, 1993.

Answer 20

a. Your patient's mutation is in the intron right next to the exon. It is certainly a splicing defect between exon 2 and intron 2. Normally, you would splice exon 1 to exon 2 to exon 3. In your patient, however, you have a cDNA that is 90 amino acids shorter than the normal cDNA. Ninety amino acids is the length of exon 2. It seems likely, therefore, that, in your patient, exon 1 is spliced directly to exon 3. This can be confirmed by the fact that your patient's cDNA has a sequence in which the 3' end of exon 1 is joined to the 5' end of exon 3:

CATTGTATG   GAAGAGATC
Exon 1   Exon 2

You will notice that the last three nucleotides in exon 1 will be transcribed as AUG, which is the initiation codon. It is possible that the gene product in your patient is translated starting here, in which case the hormone will be synthesized without the signal sequence. Without the signal sequence, the hormone will not be secreted.

b. A disease of this sort, in which there is a mutation that inactivates a protein, is likely to be recessive in the heterozygote, because a heterozygote will presumably have one functional protein. However, if the parents are closely related, then it is possible that each are carriers and hence that some of their children will be homozygous and thereby have the disease.

Your patient has AUTOSOMAL RECESSIVE HYPOPARATHYROIDISM.

REFERENCES

Parkinson, D. B., and Thakker, R. V. A donor splice site mutation in the parathyroid hormone gene is associated with autosomal recessive hypoparathyroidism. *Nat. Genet.* 1: 149, 1992.

CHAPTER 7

The Blood

Problem 21

Your patient has low levels of neutrophils and platelets as well as an autoimmune hemolytic anemia. You find that he has a mutation in his Fas gene. The alteration is in the "death domain" of the gene product. A portion of the cDNA sequence is shown here and compared to that of a normal person:

Normal person: AAAGCCAATCTTTGTACTTTGT...ACAAACTTCATCAAGAGTAAA...
Your patient: AAAGCCAATCTTTGTACTTTGTACAAACTTCATCAAGAGTAAA...

When you incubate your patient's lymphocytes with a monoclonal antibody to Fas, no apoptosis occurs, whereas 65% of the lymphocytes from a normal person undergo apoptosis in this experiment.

a. What type of mutation does your patient have and what is its consequence on the structure of the protein? What are the C-terminal 13 amino acids in your patient's Fas?

b. How does the mutation lead to the disease?

Problem 22

There are three subspecies of *Trypanosoma brucei*. These are *T. brucei gambiense, T. brucei rhodesiense,* and *T. brucei brucei*. The first two cause African sleeping sickness. The third causes a disease in animals called nagana. Morphologically, the three subspecies are apparently identical, but humans are resistant to the third species. The factor accounting for the resistance is called trypanosome lytic factor (TLF), which is a type of high-density lipoprotein (HDL). TLF contains three kinds of apolipoprotein of 45, 36, and 13.5 kD. The 45-kD subunit is apparently identical to a protein called paraoxonase-arylesterase, the 36-kD subunit to the β subunit of haptoglobin and haptoglobin-related protein, and the 13.5-kD subunit to the α subunit of haptoglobin-related protein. (Haptoglobin and haptoglobin-related protein both have the same β subunit). TLF has high peroxidase activity but only at low pH (such as pH 4). When you mix TLF with *T. brucei brucei,* you find that you can get the cells to lyse; however, addition of catalase inhibits the activity of TLF.

Speculate on how TLF kills *T. brucei brucei.*

Problem 23

Your patient has hypertension. You put her on captopril. Captopril works by affecting two pathways. Describe each pathway and the two factors whose metabolism is directly affected by captopril.

Problem 24

Your patient has a tendency to form blood clots in the veins of his legs. His father and grandfather both died suddenly of pulmonary embolism. You have purified his Factor V gene and sequenced it. You find an abnormality, shown here:

Codon number:	505	506	507
Normal person:	CGG	CGA	GGG
Your patient:	CGG	CAA	GGG

When you test the ability of his purified factor V to participate in blood coagulation, you find that its activity is perfectly normal.

Identify the mutation and explain how it leads to the symptoms.

Problem 25

Your patient has frequent hemorrhaging, particularly in his nose and his gastrointestinal system. He has some pulmonary venous malformations. He also has frequent migraine headaches. You find that he has an altered protein. In normal persons this protein, expressed in endothelial cells, binds very well to TGF-β, but the protein from your patient binds poorly to TGF-β. The nucleotide sequence of a portion of the protein is shown here both for a normal person and for your patient:

Codon number:	820	821	822	823	824	825	826
Normal person:	ACT	GGA	GAA	TAC	TCC	TTC	AAG
Your patient:	ACT	GGA	GAA	TAG	TCC	TTC	AAG

a. How would the mutation affect the observed phenotype?

b. We produce other proteins (such as β-glycan) capable of binding TGF-β. Why does a mutation in this particular protein cause a disease?

Problem 26

For much of her life your patient has suffered from repeated bacterial infections. You find that her blood neutrophil count is very low, less than 200 neutrophils per cubic millimeter. Some of your cancer patients who have low neutrophil counts following chemotherapy have responded to treatment with granulocyte-colony-stimulating factor (G-CSF). Accordingly, you start your patient on a treatment with G-CSF and she responds. Her neutrophil count rises to 6000 per cubic millimeter and her bacterial infections at first cease. Unfortunately, this is not entirely the response you want, since many of the neutrophils are immature. Your patient has developed acute myeloid leukemia and dies one year after you started treating her.

You have obtained some bone marrow cells from your patient and do an experiment in which you culture them and measure the number of granulocytes that develop as a result of treatment with various growth factors. You also culture some bone marrow cells from a normal individual for purposes of comparison. The results are shown below:

Subject	Growth Factor Added	Number of Granulocyte Colonies Formed
Normal person	Interleukin-3	0
	GM-CSF	0
	G-CSF	150
Your patient	Interleukin-3	0
	GM-CSF	0
	G-CSF	7

Note: GM-CSF stands for granulocyte/macrophage-colony-stimulating factor.

Further analysis shows that your patient has an altered protein. The alteration is shown here:

Codon number:	724	725	726	727	728	729	730	731	732	733
Normal person:	AGC	GAT	CAG	GTC	CTT	TAT	GGG	CAG	CTG	CTG
Your patient:	AGC	GAT	CAG	GTC	CTT	TAT	GGG	TAG	CTG	CTG

You do another experiment in which you clone the gene from your patient and from a normal individual into mouse myeloid cells and examine their response to G-CSF after 8 days in culture. Here are the results.

Genes Cloned	Number of Cells
Normal person's	60,000
Your patient's	100,000,000
Your patient's + normal person's	100,000,000

a. What protein is altered in your patient?

b. Why does the mutation cause the disease?

c. How could your treatment have given rise to your patient's leukemia?

d. What is the significance of the observation that the cells carrying both the normal and mutated gene are no different in their response to G-CSF than cells carrying the mutated gene alone?

Answer 21

a. Your patient has a deletion in his Fas gene. The deletion causes a STOP codon to appear and prematurely terminate the polypeptide.

Normal person: AAAGCCAATCTTTGTACTTTGT...ACAAACTTCATCAAGAGTAAA...
Your patient: AAAGCCAATCTTTGTACTTTGT ACAAACTTCATCAAGAGTAAA...

Normal person's DNA:	AAA GCC AAT CTT TGT ACT TTG T...
Normal person's RNA:	AAA GCC AAUCUU UGU ACU UUG U...
Normal person's protein:	Lys Ala Asn Leu Cys Thr Leu
Your patient's DNA:	AAA GCC AAT CTT TGT ACT TTG TAC AAA CTT CAT CAA GAG TAA A..
Your patient's RNA:	AAA GCC AAUCUU UGU ACU UUG UAC AAA CUU CAU CAA GAG UAA A...
Your patient's protein:	Lys Ala Asn Leu Cys Thr Leu Tyr Lys Leu His Gln Glu STOP

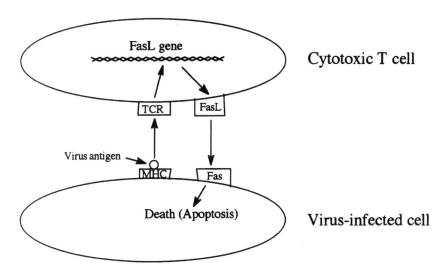

FIGURE A21. **Fas can induce apoptosis in a virus-infected cell.** The virus-infected cell (bottom) produces a portion of the virus antigen, which is then presented by the major histocompatibility complex (MHC) on the surface of the virus-infected cell. The antigen–MHC complex is then recognized by the T-cell receptor (TCR), located on the surface of the T cell (top). This binding then causes the TCR to send a transcriptional activation signal to the T-cell nucleus, causing the transcription of the FasL (Fas ligand) gene. This then leads to the expression of the FasL protein on the surface of the T cell. When FasL interacts with Fas, which is already expressed on the virus-infected cell, Fas is stimulated to start the series of events that leads to apoptosis.

b. The Fas protein is a mediator of apoptosis, programmed cell death. If it does not work well, there will be too many lymphocytes and he will have an autoimmune disease. Apoptosis is a process whereby, often in response to a signal, a cell will go through a program of self-destruction. It is a highly useful process in that it can rid the body of cells that turn cancerous or that become infected with viruses. Fas can induce apoptosis in various situations. Figure A21-1 shows how Fas can be triggered to destroy a virus-infected cell.

Your patient has LYMPHOPROLIFERATIVE DISORDER.

REFERENCES

Cohen, J. J., Duke, R. C., Fadok, V. A., and Sellins, K. S. Apoptosis and programmed cell death in immunity. *Annu. Rev. Immunol.* 10: 267, 1992.

Hale, A. J., Smith, C. A., Sutherland, L. C., Stoneman, V. E. A., Longthorne, V. L.,
Culhane, A. C., and Williams, G. T. Apoptosis: Molecular regulation of cell
death. *Eur. J. Biochem.* 236: 1, 1996.

Nagata, S., and Golstein, P. The Fas death factor. *Science* 267: 1449, 1995.

Rieux-Laucat, F., Le Deist, F., Hivroz, C., Roberts, I. A. G., Debatin, K. M., Fischer,
A., de Villartay, J. P. Mutations in Fas associated with human lymphoproliferative syndrome and autoimmunity. *Science* 268: 1347, 1995.

Answer 22

TLF has two kinds of activity: the paraoxonase-arylesterase and a
peroxidase activity. Since it contains haptoglobin-related protein, it

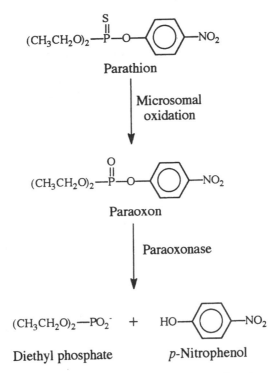

FIGURE A22-1. **Paraoxonase pathway.** The pathway is used to degrade the insecti-
cide parathion.

is likely that it can bind to hemoglobin as does haptoglobin. *T. brucei brucei* will cause an erythrocyte to lyse; it will ingest the hemoglobin and any other protein that binds it, such as TLF. When the TLF reaches the lysosomes of the trypanosome, the low pH activates the peroxidase activity, which then disrupts the lysosomal membrane. This in turn causes the lysosomal enzymes to be released into the cytosol and, in effect, the trypanosome digests itself.

REFERENCES

Furlong, C. E., Costa, L. G., Hassett, C., Richter, R. J., Sundstrom, J. A., Adler, D. A., Disteche, C. M., Omiecinski, C. J., Chapline, C., Crabb, J. W., and Humbert, R. Human and rabbit paraoxonases: Purification, cloning, sequencing, mapping and role of polymorphism in organophosphate detoxification. *Chem. Biol. Interact.* 87: 35, 1993.

Smith, A. B., Esko, J. D., and Hajduk, S. L. Killing of trypanosomes by the human haptoglobin-related protein. *Science* 268: 284, 1995.

Answer 23

Captopril (Fig. A23-1) inhibits two types of enzyme. One is *angiotensin-converting enzyme* (ACE), which converts angiotensin I to angiotensin II. The other enzyme is *kininase II*, which converts bradykinin to inactive peptides and amino acids. The two pathways (shown in Figure A23-2) are as follows:

Kininogen → bradykinin → inactive peptides
Angiotensinogen → angiotensin I → angiotensin II → inactive peptides

Angiotensin II works to raise blood pressure. By inhibiting its formation, blood pressure is reduced. Bradykinin stimulates the

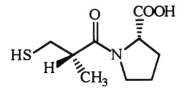

FIGURE A23-1. **Structure of captopril.**

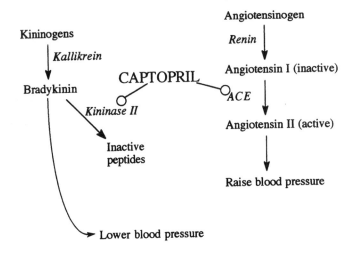

—○ = Inhibits

ACE = Angiotensin converting enzyme

FIGURE A23-2. **How captopril acts to lower blood pressure.** Captopril inhibits two proteolytic enzymes: kininase II and ACE. The inhibition of kininase II prevents bradykinin from being degraded and thereby raises its concentration. Angiotensin II is a potent hypertensive agent. Captopril's inhibition of ACE blocks angiotensin II synthesis, thereby lessening the latter's hypertensive effect.

synthesis of PGI_2 and PGE_2, which lower blood pressure. By inhibiting the degradation of bradykinin, we again lower the blood pressure.

REFERENCES

Shapiro, A. P. Inhibitors of angiotensin-converting enzyme in the management of hypertension. R. H. Glew and S. P. Peters (Eds.). *Clinical Studies in Medical Biochemistry.* New York: Oxford University Press, 1987, pp. 241–252.

Answer 24

The mutation is analyzed as follows:

Codon number:	505	506	507
Normal person's DNA:	CGG	CGA	GGG
Normal person's RNA:	CGG	CGA	GGG
Normal person's protein:	Arg	Arg	Gly
Your patient's DNA:	CGG	CAA	GGG
Your patient's RNA:	CGG	CAA	GGG
Your patient's protein:	Arg	Gln	Gly

Your patient has a glutamine at position 506 instead of an arginine. This is the position at which factor V is cleaved by activated protein C as part of the regulation of blood coagulation. Since factor V acts to speed up coagulation, its inactivation is an important part of regulating coagulation. Activated protein C is a proteolytic enzyme which does this. It also cleaves and inactivates factor VIII. Your patient's factor V will not be cleaved by activated protein C and, hence, will remain active much longer, leading to excessive clotting. This particular mutation may account for about 25% of the cases of venous thrombosis.

Your patient has VENOUS THROMBOSIS.

REFERENCES

Bertina, R. M., Koeleman, B. P. C., Koster, T., Rosendaal, F. R., Dirven, R. J., de Ronde, H., van der Velden, P. A., and Reitsma, P. H. Mutation in blood coagulation factor V associated with resistance to activated protein C. *Nature* 369: 64, 1994.

Majerus, P. W. Bad blood by mutation. *Nature* 369: 14, 1994.

Answer 25

a. The mutation is analyzed below:

Codon number:	820	821	822	823	824	825	826
Normal person's DNA:	ACT	GGA	GAA	TAC	TCC	TTC	AAG
Normal person's RNA:	ACU	GGA	GAA	UAC	UCC	UUC	AAG
Normal person's protein:	Thr	Glu	Glu	Tyr	Ser	Phe	Lys
Your patient's DNA:	ACT	GGA	GAA	TAG	TCC	TTC	AAG
Your patient's RNA:	ACU	GGA	GAA	UAG	UCC	UUC	AAG
Your patient's protein:	Thr	Gly	Glu	STOP			

Your patient has a nonsense mutation, which causes premature termination. He probably produces a nonfunctional protein. TGF-β (transforming growth factor β) is a potent angiogenic signal, which helps to determine the morphology of growing blood vessels. It stimulates endothelial cells to produce matrix proteins including the basement membrane. If your patient lacks the binding protein, the endothelial cells will not form correctly and the blood vessels will be fragile, leading to frequent hemorrhaging. In addition, the blood vessels will be malformed.

b. The protein we are discussing has been named *endoglin*. It forms a complex with TGF-β and two receptors called RI and RII. The complex then stimulates the endothelial cells. Many other cells in our bodies produce another protein, called β-glycan, which is very similar to endoglin. The difference is that β-glycan binds all three isoforms of TGF-β and endoglin binds only TGF-β1 and TGF-β3. In many cells, β-glycan could compensate for defective endoglin. However, endothelial cells make very little β-glycan, hence they are very vulnerable to mutations in endoglin.

Your patient has HEREDITARY HEMORRHAGIC TELANGIECTASIA TYPE I.

REFERENCES

McAllister, K. A. Grogg, K. M., Johnson, D. W., Gallione, C. J., Baldwin, M. A., Jackson, C. E., Helmbold, E. A., Markel, D. S., Mckinnon, W. C., Murrell, J.,

McCormick, M. K., Pericak-Vance, M. A., Heutink, P., Oostra, B. A., Haitjema, T., Westerman, C. J. J., Porteous, M. E., Guttmacher, A. E., Letarte, M., and Marchuk, D. A. Endoglin, a TGF-β binding protein of endothelial cells, is the gene for hereditary haemorrhagic telangiectasia type 1. *Nat. Genet.* 8: 345, 1994.

Answer 26

a. Your patient's bone marrow cells respond very poorly to G-CSF. This suggests that the defective protein is a receptor. In fact, it is *granulocyte-colony-stimulating factor receptor.*

b. First, analyze the mutation:

Codon number:	724	725	726	727	728	729	730	731	732	733
Normal person's										
DNA:	AGC	GAT	CAG	GTC	CTT	TAT	GGG	CAG	CTG	CTG
RNA:	AGC	GAU	CAG	GUC	CUU	UAU	GGG	CAG	CUG	CUG
Protein:	Ser	Asp	Gln	Val	Leu	Tyr	Gly	Gln	Leu	Leu
Your patient's										
DNA:	AGC	GAT	CAG	GTC	CTT	TAT	GGG	TAG	CTG	CTG
RNA:	AGC	GAU	CAG	GUC	CUU	UAU	GGG	UAG	CUG	CUG
Protein:	Ser	Asp	Gln	Val	Leu	Tyr	Gly	STOP		

In general, membrane-bound receptors such as this have three functional domains. These are: (1) the extracellular domain to which the agonist binds, in this case G-CSF; (2) a transmembrane domain; and (3) an intracellular or cytoplasmic domain that will initiate the response to the agonist. In the case of G-CSF receptor, the extracellular domain consists of the first 604 residues, while the transmembrane domain includes residues 605 to 630, and the intracellular domain is residues 631 to 813. Your patient's mutation, at position 731, is in the intracellular domain. Your patient's protein is lacking a substantial portion of the C-terminal cytoplasmic domain. It is not surprising that it is unable to initiate the response to G-CSF. A normal receptor would have responded to G-CSF by inducing maturation of the cells into granulocytes, but, in your patient's case, with a defective cytoplasmic domain, this cannot happen.

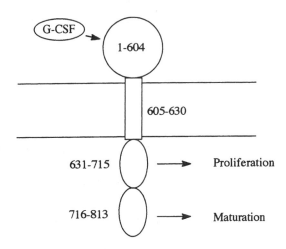

NORMAL PERSON

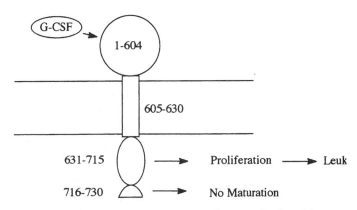

YOUR PATIENT

FIGURE A26-1. **Action of the G-CSF receptor in a normal person (top) and in your patient (bottom).** The key feature of this receptor is that it has two cytoplasmic domains, one to mediate cell proliferation and the other to mediate cell maturation. In a normal person, G-CSF will stimulate both effects, leading to normal granulocyte production. In your patient, G-CSF will stimulate only proliferation. The large number of immature cells leads to leukemia.

c. In reality, the G-CSF receptor is somewhat more complex than other receptors. Its cytoplasmic domain is actually divided into two smaller domains. The N terminal of these two domains responds to G-CSF by initiating proliferation (cell multiplication) without maturation; the other domain responds by initiating cell maturation. Since your patient's mutation is in the second of these two domains, G-CSF will be unable to induce maturation; however, it will have no trouble inducing proliferation. Proliferation of excess immature cells is leukemia.

d. The table shows that the presence of the mutant gene overwhelms the presence of the normal gene. This is because the G-CSF receptor, when in the presence of G-CSF, forms a tetramer. Thus, most of the G-CSF receptors in your patient's bone marrow cells will contain at least one mutant subunit. This may be enough for them to function improperly.

Your patient has SEVERE CONGENITAL NEUTROPENIA.

REFERENCES

Dong, F., van Buitenen, C., Pouwels, K., Hoefsloot, L. H., Löwenberg, B., and Touw, I. P., Distinct cytoplasmic regions of the human granulocyte colony-stimulating factor receptor involved in induction of proliferation and maturation. *Mol. Cell. Biol.* 13: 7774, 1993.

Dong, F., Hoefsloot, L. H., Schelen, A. M., Broeders, L. C.A. M., Meijer, Y., Veerman, A. J. P., Touw, I. P., and Löwenberg, B., Identification of a nonsense mutation in the granulocyte-colony-stimulating factor receptor in severe congenital neutropenia. *Proc. Natl. Acad. Sci. USA* 91: 4480, 1994.

Dong, F. D., Brynes, R. K., Tidow, N., Welte, K., Löwenberg, B., and Touw, I. P. Mutations in the gene for the granulocyte colony-stimulating-factor receptor in patients with acute myeloid leukemia preceded by severe congenital neutropenia. *N. Engl. J. Med.* 333: 487, 1995.

Fukunaga, R., Seto, Y., Mizushima, S., and Nagata, S. Three different mRNAs encoding human granulocyte colony-stimulating factor receptor. *Proc. Natl. Acad. Sci. USA* 87: 8702, 1990.

Fukunaga, R., Ishizaka-Ikeda, E., and Nagata, S. Growth and differentiation signals mediated by different regions in the cytoplasmic domain of granulocyte colony-stimulating factor receptor. *Cell* 74: 1079, 1993.

Hiraoka, O., Anaguchi, H., and Ota, Y. Evidence for the ligand-induced conversion from a dimer to a tetramer of the granulocyte colony-stimulating factor receptor. *FEBS Lett.* 256: 255, 1994.

Naparstek, E. Granulocyte colony-stimulating factor, congenital neutropenia, and acute myeloid leukemia. *N. Engl. J. Med.* 333: 516, 1995.

Ziegler, S. F., Bird, T. A., Morella, K. K., Mosley, B., Gearing, D. P., and Baumann, H. Distinct regions of the human granulocyte-colony-stimulating factor receptor cytoplasmic domain are required for proliferation and gene induction. *Mol. Cell. Biol.* 13: 2384, 1993.

CHAPTER 8

The Immune System

Problem 27

Your patient is a 1-year-old girl who has been very sick for her entire life. She often gets infections. Your patient's total T-cell count is normal, but CD8$^+$ cells are much fewer than normal. You isolated her CD4$^+$ T cells and observed that they do not respond to phytohemagglutinin or concanavalin A. In contrast, normal cells do proliferate. However, if you give your patient's cells phorbol esters and calcium ionophores, they proliferate normally.

You culture your patient's CD4$^+$ cells and treat with a monoclonal antibody to CD3. You find no increase in cytoplasmic calcium in those cells whereas the same cells from a normal person show a great increase in calcium. You also treat the cells with a combination of biotinylated anti-CD3 and anti-CD4 and add avidin. You then lyse the cells and analyze them on a gel with an antibody to phosphotyrosine. You find that your patient's cells are unable to make proteins that react with the antibody to phosphotyrosine. The normal cells made several such proteins.

You find a protein that is altered in your patient. Here is a portion of the sequence:

Codon number: 515   516   517   518   519   520   521
Normal person: AAG TTC TCC AGC CGC AGC GAT
Your patient: AAG TTC TCC AGA CGC AGC GAT

The region shown above tends to be highly conserved in proteins of this family.

a. What is the likely function of the defective protein?

b. How does the defect lead to the disease?

Problem 28

There have been reports that marijuana has some immunosuppressive properties. Recently, a protein has been discovered that may mediate the immunosuppressive effects of marijuana.

a. What is this protein and in what cell type is it likely to be located?

b. Is it able to bind to anandamide?

c. If a person had a mutation in this protein such that it was no longer affected by marijuana, would that person still be able to get "high" when he smoked marijuana? Why or why not?

Problem 29

Your patient is severely allergic to many pollens and to dust mites. You have cloned and sequenced the gene for protein FcεR1-β. Your analysis of the sequence suggests that this is a membrane protein. You find that the sequence of this gene in your patient differs at two positions from that of another individual who is not allergic:

Codon number:	181	182	183
Normal person:	ATT	GTA	GTG
Your patient:	TTG	GTA	TTG

The region shown above is in a transmembrane segment.

a. What is the function of FcεR1-β?

b. How might the alteration cause the allergic symptoms?

Problem 30

Your patient is a 1-year-old girl who repeatedly has serious infections. She has had diarrhea, meningitis, and various abscesses. You do many tests on her immune system and the only oddity you find is that her phagocytes do not attack yeast cells. She has a mutation in the gene coding for a certain protein. In this protein, a glycine at position 54 is replaced by an aspartic acid. When you clone and express your patient's protein, you find that it is unable to bind to mannan or to mannose.

You have an antibody to this protein and you do two assays. In one, you do an ELISA to measure the serum levels of this protein; here you find that your patient's serum has a concentration of this protein of 5 ng/ml, whereas a normal person has about 1630 ng/ml. You then subject serum from your patient and from a normal person to polyacrylamide gel electrophoresis in the presence of sodium dodecyl sulfate. On the same gel you also run some of the recombinant protein as well as a series of proteins of known molecular weight. After the gel is done, you do a Western blot on it with the antibody. You observe that, in each sample, multiple bands show up. In the serum from a normal person as well as in the sample of recombinant protein, you find that the bands range in molecular weight from 70 to 700 kD, with the major bands at 200, 300, and 400 kD. In the serum from your patient, however, the bands range in molecular weight from 70 to 400 kD, with the major band at 120 kD.

a. What is the defective protein?

b. How does the mutation lead to the disease?

Answer 27

a. The defective protein is likely to be a tyrosine kinase. In fact, it is called *ZAP-70*. It is the T-cell receptor. When the T-cell receptor meets its preferred ligand, it activates the tyrosine kinase, which in turn activates a phospholipase C whose activity leads to the entry of calcium into the cell. This leads to the proliferation of the cell and the immune response.

b. The mutation is analyzed here:

Codon number:	515	516	517	518	519	520	521
Normal person's DNA:	AAG	TTC	TCC	AGC	CGC	AGC	GAT
Normal person's RNA:	AAG	UUC	UCC	AGC	CGC	AGC	GAU
Normal person's protein:	Lys	Phe	Ser	Ser	Arg	Ser	Asp
Your patient's DNA:	AAG	TTC	TCC	AGA	CGC	AGC	GAT
Your patient's RNA:	AAG	UUC	UCC	AGA	CGC	AGC	GAU
Your patient's protein:	Lys	Phe	Ser	Arg	Arg	Ser	Asp

Your patient has an arginine at position 518 instead of a serine. Because this is a highly conserved region, it is likely that any change would be deleterious, particularly one that substitutes a large, positively charged residue for a small uncharged one. Inability of ZAP-70 to work means that T cells will not respond to signals and the immune response will be compromised, leading to frequent infections.

Your patient has SEVERE COMBINED IMMUNODEFICIENCY.

REFERENCES

Chan, A. C., Kadlecek, T. A., Elder, M. E., Filipovich, A. H., Kuo, W.-L., Iwashima, M., Parslow, T. G., and Weiss, A. ZAP-70 deficiency in an autosomal recessive form of severe combined immunodeficiency. *Science* 264: 1599, 1994.

Elder, M. E., Lin, D., Clever, J., Chan, A. C., Hope, T. J., Weiss, A., and Parslow, T. G. Human severe combined immunodeficiency due to a defect in ZAP-70, a T cell tyrosine kinase. *Science* 264: 1596, 1994.

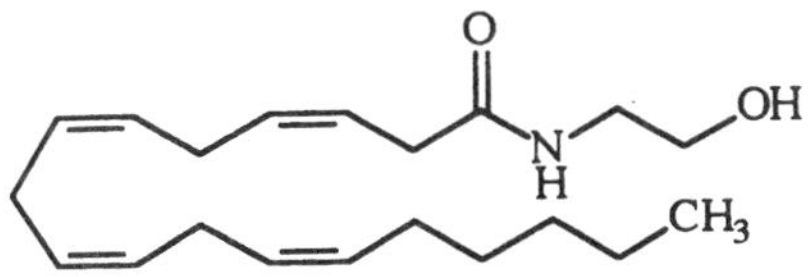

FIGURE A28-1. **Structure of anandamide.** This compound, as can be gathered from its structure, is a derivative of arachidonic acid. It gets its name from the Sanskrit word "ananda," which means "internal bliss."

Answer 28

a. The active ingredient in marijuana is $\triangle^9$-tetrahydrocannabinol. There is a receptor for this compound in macrophages and, in fact, incubation with $\triangle^9$-tetrahydrocannabinol inhibits their spreading and phagocytosis *in vitro*.

b. The macrophage receptor binds to anandamide (Fig. A28-1), the endogenous ligand for cannabinoid receptors.

c. The brain receptor for cannabinoids appears to be a very different protein from the macrophage receptor. Thus, a mutation in the macrophage protein should not affect the brain receptor and the person with the mutation should still be able to get "high" from smoking marijuana.

REFERENCES

Barinaga, M. Pot, heroin unlock new areas for neuroscience. *Science* 258: 1882, 1992.

Lopez-Ceperom, M., Friedman, M., Klein, T., and Friedman, H. Tetrahydrocannabinol-induced suppression of macrophage spreading and phagocytic activity in vitro. *J. Leukoc. Biol.* 39: 679, 1986.

Munro, S., Thomas, K. L., and Abu-Shaar, M. Molecular characterization of a peripheral receptor for cannabinoids. *Nature* 365: 61, 1993.

Answer 29

a. The protein FcϵR1-β is the immunoglobulin E (IgE) receptor. It is located in mast cells and other types of cell. IgE binds to it

and, when the IgE binds to its antigen, the receptor initiates the release of the allergy-mediating factors.

b. The mutation is analyzed as follows:

Codon number:	181	182	183
Normal person's DNA:	ATT	GTA	GTG
Normal person's RNA:	AUU	GUA	GUG
Normal person's protein:	Ilu	Val	Val
Your patient's DNA:	TTG	GTA	TTG
Your patient's RNA:	UUG	GUA	UUG
Your patient's protein:	Leu	Val	Leu

The changes in your patient's sequence include a leucine at position 181 instead of isoleucine and a leucine at position 183 instead
of valine. The two changes replace hydrophobic acids with other
hydrophobic acids and, in many proteins, might be expected to be
relatively neutral in their effects, but in a transmembrane domain,
they may have bigger effects. It is possible that the IgE receptor in
your patient is set up so that it transmits signals more easily, or
transmits weaker signals. In short, your patient may react to certain antigens more strongly than other people would.

Your patient has ATOPY.

REFERENCES

Shirakawa, T., Li, A., Dubowitz, M., Dekker, J. W., Shaw, A. E., Faux, J. A., Ra, C.,
Cookson, W. O. C. M., and Hopkin, J. M. Association between atopy and vari-
ants of the β subunit of the high-affinity immunoglobulin E receptor. *Nat.
Genet.* 7: 125, 1994.

Answer 30

a. The defective protein is called mannose-binding protein. Its
job apparently is to bind to mannose residues in yeast cell walls or
in certain bacterial cell envelopes and to initiate the classical com-

plement pathway. This protein therefore provides a kind of automatic immunity to certain pathogens, a type of immunity that does not require an antibody. Without mannose-binding protein, we become very susceptible to infections. Even if we subsequently develop antibody-mediated immunity to the pathogen, our initial infection is a very serious one.

Yeast cell walls are made of mannans, which contain large numbers of mannose residues. Mannans are in essence glycoproteins in which an oligosaccharide subunit consisting of mannose residues is attached to an asparagine residue via a bridge of two residues of N-acetylglucosamine. A large number of oligosaccharide subunits are involved. In the cases of the yeasts *Saccharomyces kluyveri* and the pathogenic *Candida tropicalis*, the oligosaccharide subunits are thought to consist of 27 and 42 mannose residues, respectively.

b. The mannose-binding protein is formed from a single polypeptide chain that contains a collagen-like N-terminal domain where three of these chains join to form a triple helix; the chains are also held together by disulfide bonds. The entire mannose-binding protein is then formed of 2 to 6 of these trimers. Glycine 52 is at one of the sites in the triple-helical collagen-like domain where the side chain is supposed to project in toward the middle of the triple helix. This occurs at every third position, all of which are glycines in this region. Since glycine has essentially no side chain, it is the perfect, in fact the only, acceptable residue at this position. Replacing the glycine with an aspartic acid weakens the triple helix. Clearly your patient has very little of the mannose-binding protein in her serum. The results of the Western blot are very illuminating. In the serum from a normal person, the protein forms a series of oligomers; however, the recombinant mutant protein also forms the same series of oligomers. However, in your patient's serum, the oligomers are much smaller. This suggests that, in your patient's serum, the concentrations of the subunits are much lower and, hence, oligomerization is inhibited. The probable explanation is that the mutation alters the secondary structure of the protein in such a way as to make the protein more susceptible to degradation.

REFERENCES

Kobayashi, H., Matsuda, K., Ikeda, T., Suzuki, M., Takahashi, S. I., Suzuki, A., Shibata, N., and Suzuki, S. Structures of cell wall mannans of pathogenic *Candida tropicalis* IFO 0199 and IFO 1647 yeast strains. *Infect. Immun.* 62: 615, 1994.

Lipscombe, R. J., Sumiya, M., Summerfield, J. A., and Turner, M. W. Distinct physicochemical characteristics of human mannose binding protein expressed by individuals of differing phenotype. *Immunology* 85: 660, 1995.

Shibata, N., Kojima, C., Satoh, Y., Satoh, R., Suzuki, A., Kobayashi, H., and Suzuki, S. Structural study of a cell-wall mannan of *Saccharomyces kluyveri* IFO 1685 strain. Presence of a branched side chain and β-1,2-linkage. *Eur. J. Biochem.* 217: 1, 1993.

Summerfield, J. A., Ryder, S., Sumiya, M., Thursz, M., Gorchein, A., Monteil, M. A., and Turner, M. W. Mannose-binding protein gene mutations associated with unusual and severe infections in adults. *Lancet* 345: 886, 1995.

Thompson, C. Protein proves to be a key link in innate immunity. *Science* 269: 301, 1995.

CHAPTER 9

Infections

Problem 31

Diphtheria toxin works by ADP ribosylating the elongation factor EF-2.

a. How is diphtheria toxin made and processed?

b. What is special about the residue on EF-2, which is the target for diphtheria toxin?

c. How is that residue formed?

d. Would you expect diphtheria toxin to target elongation factor in mitochondria? Why or why not?

Problem 32

a. What protein or proteins are the target for tetanus toxin?

b. What is the normal function of that protein or proteins?

Problem 33

Your patient is about to undertake an archaeological expedition to the border region of Thailand and Cambodia. She has heard that the strain, found in that area, of the mosquito-borne malarial parasite *Plasmodium falciparum,* is resistant to all known antimalarial drugs. The reason for this is that during the political upheavals of the last two decades, very large numbers of refugees, soldiers, guerillas, and others traversed the area, overdosing themselves prophylactically with various antimalarial drugs, until, through natural selection, the parasites became completely resistant. She asks you, therefore, if there is any chance of a malarial vaccine being developed sometime soon. You tell her that scientists are trying to develop a vaccine against *P. falciparum* erythrocyte membrane protein 1.

a. What is this protein and why is it an attractive target for a malarial vaccine?

b. What is the major obstacle to creating a vaccine against this protein?

Answer 31

a. Diphtheria toxin is made in the bacterium *Corynebacterium diphtheriae*. The gene for it is actually encoded by a bacteriophage (phage b), which infects the bacterium. The toxin is made as a single precursor polypeptide with no activity and with two intrachain disulfides. Upon infection, the toxin binds to a receptor on the membrane of a target cell. The toxin then enters the endosomes where it is cleaved and reduced and the active enzyme released into the cytoplasm.

b. The target residue for diphtheria is a modified histidine called 2-[3-carboxyamido-3-(trimethylamino)propyl]histidine, or *diphthamide*. It is this residue that becomes ADP ribosylated (Fig. A31-2). It is thought that this modification confers some heat resistance on EF-2.

c. The pathway for diphthamide synthesis in yeast is as follows (Fig. A31-1):

Histidine → 2-[3-amino-3-carboxypropyl]histidine → diphthine → diphthamide

d. Mitochondrial elongation factor resembles eubacterial elongation factors in that it lacks the histidine that is turned into diphthamide. Presumably, the bacteria that synthesize diphthamide must be resistant to it as well. You would not expect mitochondria to be sensitive to diphtheria toxin.

REFERENCES

Barker, C., Makris, A., Patriotis, C., Bear, S. E., and Tsichlis, P. N. Identification of the gene encoding the mitochondrial elongation factor G in mammals. *Nucl. Acids Res.* 21: 2641, 1993.

Dunlop, P. C., and Bodley, J. W. Biosynthetic labeling of diphthamide in *Saccharomyces cerevisiae*. *J. Biol. Chem.* 258: 4754, 1983.

Jagus, R., Dowling, J. N., Moss, J., and Vaughan, M. Bacterial toxins: diphtheria and cholera. R. H. Glew, and S. P. Peters, (Eds.). *Clinical Studies in Medical Biochemistry.* New York: Oxford University Press, 1987, pp. 52–65.

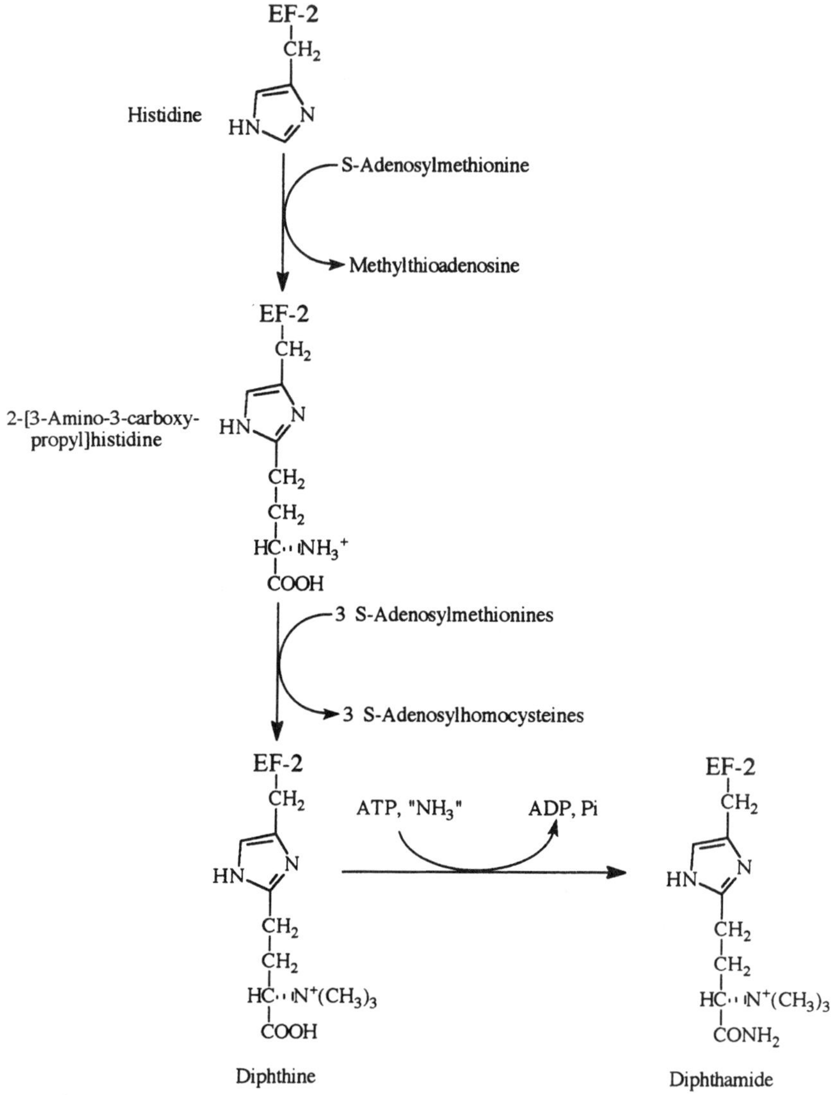

FIGURE A31-1. **Pathway of diphthamide synthesis.**

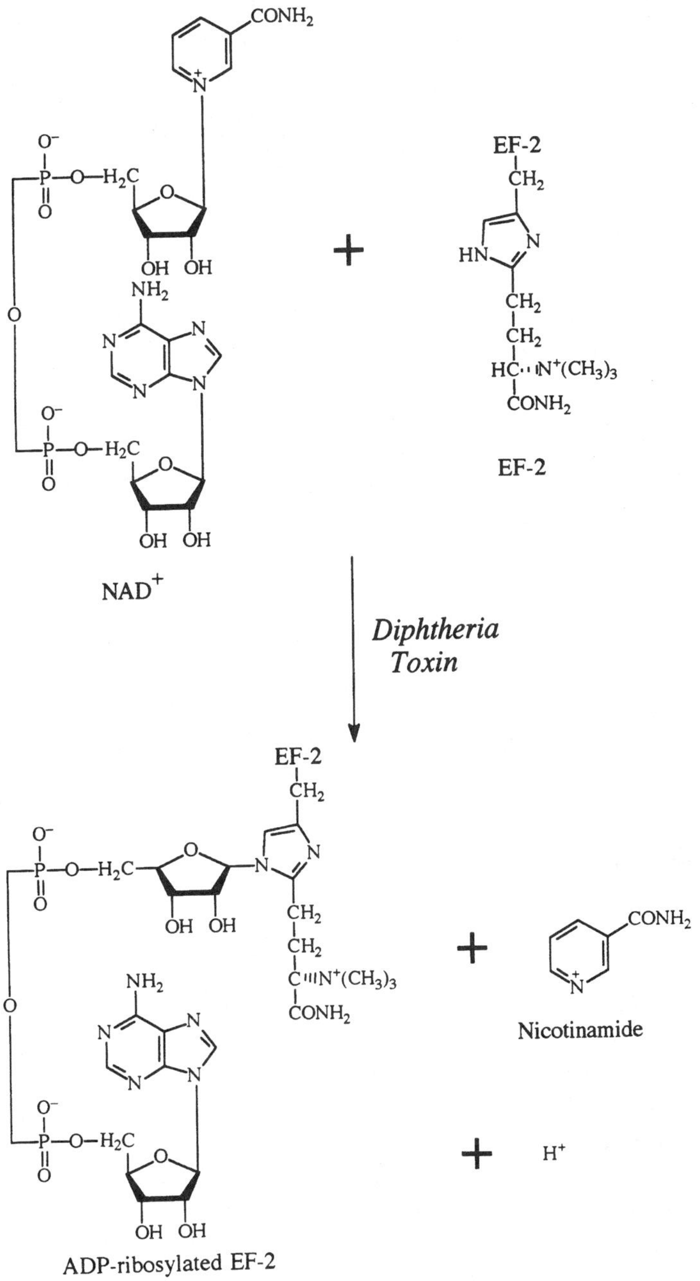

FIGURE A31-2. **ADP ribosylation of elongation factor 2 (EF-2) by diphtheria toxin reacting with diphthamide.**

Kimata, Y., and Kohno, K. Elongation factor 2 mutants deficient in diphthamide formation show temperature-sensitive cell growth. *J. Biol. Chem.* 269: 13497, 1994.

Mattheakis, L. C., Sor, F., and Collier, R. J. Diphthamide synthesis in *Saccharomyces cerevisiae*: Structure of the *DPH2* gene. *Gene* 132: 149, 1993.

Answer 32

a. Tetanus toxin is an endopeptidase that cleaves two similar proteins: *synaptobrevin II* and *cellubrevin*.

b. Synaptobrevin II is found at the synapse. It appears to play a critical role in fusion of the synaptic vesicle with the membrane and hence with release of neurotransmitters. Cellubrevin is much more widespread, and it may have a similar function in vesicle fusion.

REFERENCES

McMahon, H. T., Ushkaryov, Y. A., Edelmann, L., Link, E., Binz, T. Niemann, H., Jahn, R., and Südhof, T. C. Cellubrevin is a ubiquitous tetanus-toxin substrate homologous to a putative synaptic vesicle fusion protein. *Nature* 364: 346, 1993.

Shiavo, G., Benfenati, F., Poulain, B., Rossetto, O., Polverino de Laureto, P., DasGupta, B. R., and Montecucco, C. Tetanus and botulinum-B neurotoxins block neurotransmitter release by proteolytic cleavage of synaptobrevin. *Nature* 359: 832, 1992.

Answer 33

a. The parasite *P. falciparum* passes much of its life cycle in the erythrocyte where it is hidden from most vaccines. However, it expresses this protein (erythrocyte membrane protein 1), which ends up in the erythrocyte membrane and mediates adhesion to thrombospondin and other adhesion molecules. It is through this protein, therefore, that the parasite causes much of its pathogenic effect. At the same time, the protein is an attractive target because, being expressed on the erythrocyte membrane, it is accessible to our immune system.

b. The chief obstacle is that *P. falciparum* keeps changing the sequence of the protein through various recombinations of a total of 50 to 150 genes. This variability makes it very difficult to find a specific target for a vaccine.

REFERENCES

Baruch, D. I., Pasloske, B. L., Singh, H. B., Bi, X., Ma, X. C., Feldman, M., Taraschi, T. F., and Howard, R. J. Cloning the *P. falciparum* gene encoding PfEMP1, a malarial variant antigen and adherence receptor on the surface of parasitized human erythrocytes. *Cell* 82: 77, 1995.

Garrett, L. *The Coming Plague: Newly Emerging Diseases in a World out of Balance.* New York: Farrar, Straus and Giroux, 1994.

Su, Z., Heatwole, V. M., Wertheimer, S. P., Guinet, F., Herrfeldt, J. A., Peterson, D. S., Ravetch, J. A., and Wellems, T. E. The large diverse gene family *var* encodes proteins involved in cytoadherence and antigenic variation of *Plasmodium falciparum*-infected erythrocytes. *Cell* 82: 89, 1995.

CHAPTER 10

The Muscles

Problem 34

Your patient began having increasing weakness in his leg and arm muscles when he was 15. He is now 25. His serum creatine kinase is elevated. You find an alteration in his gene for a calpain called CANP3. The alteration is shown here:

Codon number:	180	181	182	183	184
Normal person:	GAC	TGC	CTG	CCA	ACG
Your patient:	GAC	TGC	CAG	CCA	ACG

How might this mutation cause the disease? The answer to this question is not yet known, so some informed speculation is in order here.

Problem 35

Your patient has had gradually increasing muscle weakness. He also has cataracts and cardiac arrhythmia. His mother has similar but milder symptoms and his maternal grandmother has even milder symptoms. You have identified a major alteration in your patient's DNA. The variation appears to be an insertion into the 3' untranslated region of a protein kinase gene. The insertion begins about 177 nucleotides down from the STOP codon. The insertion consists of over 130 repeats of the sequence GCT. In that region a normal individual has anywhere from 5 to 22 GCT triplets. You observe that your patient's DNA is unable to make mRNA coding for that protein kinase.

You do the following experiment. You take the segment of DNA from your patient that contains the 130 repeats and insert it into a plasmid. You also insert the corresponding region from his mother's gene and from his grandmother's gene. You then add a preparation of histones and allow the mixture to incubate. You then examine the DNA molecules by electron microscopy. You observe that almost all of the DNA molecules have small blobs. In the control sample with only plasmids, the blobs are evenly distributed, but in the plasmids containing your patient's DNA, 48% of the blobs are in that segment, which itself only accounts for 15% of the length of the recombinant plasmid. In his mother's case, 32% of the blobs are in that segment and in his grandmother's case, 24%.

a. Speculate on how the mutation prevents the gene from being expressed.

b. Why does this disease increase in severity with each generation?

Problem 36

Your patient is a young man with severe muscle weakness. A biopsy specimen shows the presence of rod-shaped bodies in his muscles. These bodies consist largely of actin and α-actinin with some tropomyosin. You analyze the gene for his α-tropomyosin 3 and find the following:

Codon number:	2	3	4	5	6	7	8	9	10	11
Normal person:	ATG	GAG	GCC	ATC	AAG	AAA	AAG	ATG	CAG	ATG
Your patient:	ATG	GAG	GCC	ATC	AAG	AAA	AAG	ACG	CAG	ATG

a. Speculate as to how the mutation may lead to the disease.

b. How are the different forms of tropomyosin expressed?

Problem 37

Your patient has a dilated heart, but his other muscles are perfectly normal. When you examine his dystrophin gene, you notice that exon 1 and the adjacent promoter of the muscle isoform of dystrophin have been deleted. You do a skeletal muscle biopsy on your patient and on a normal individual and you measure the level of the three major dystrophin isoforms. As a comparison, you use a mouse brain. For obvious reasons, you cannot do a cardiac biopsy on your patient. Here are the results:

Tissue	Muscle Isoform	Brain Isoform	Purkinje Cell Isoform
Normal skeletal muscle	28	4	0
Normal cardiac muscle	38	22	0
Your patient's skeletal muscle	0	40	12
Mouse cerebellum	1	41	10
Mouse cerebral cortex	7	36	1

a. Why does your patient not suffer dystrophy of his skeletal muscles?

b. Why does he have any symptoms?

Feel free to speculate.

Problem 38

Your patient is a 6-month-old boy who has had severe muscular problems since birth. Even prior to his birth, his mother noted that he rarely moved. After birth, he exhibited a poor sucking reaction and cried weakly. He has a funnel chest. He is generally very weak for his age. Occasionally, however, he has major seizures. He has difficulty supporting his head. A muscle biopsy reveals that his fibers are rounded and not shaped like polygons. There is an increase in endomysial collagen.

You find that your patient has a deletion in the gene coding for laminin α2. The deletion removes base pairs 4573 to 4765.

Here is a portion of the sequence of laminin α2 in a normal individual beginning with base pair number 4565:

Codon
number: 1506 1507 1508 1509 1510 . . . 1571 1572 1573 1574 1575 1576 1577 1578 1579 1580
DNA: TGT GAA AGG TGT GCC . . . TGT GTT TTT TGT GGA GAT GAG TGC ACT GGC

How does the mutation cause the observed symptoms?

Problem 39

Your patient is a 23-year-old man who has widespread muscle weakness that began when he was 15 years old and gradually increased. He is unable to straighten out his arm at the elbow. Two years ago, cardiac problems led to implantation of a pacemaker, which saved his life. Your patient has an altered gene, part of whose sequence is shown here, compared to that for a normal individual:

Codon:	224	225	226	227	228
Normal person:	CCG	CTC	TGG	GGC	CAG
Your patient:	CCG	CTC	TAG	GGC	CAG

The normal protein consists of a single polypeptide 254 residues in length. You make a polyclonal antibody to the normal protein and use it in immunohistochemical experiments to localize the protein in various cells prepared from biopsy samples of your patient and of a normal individual. You find that in skeletal and cardiac muscles from a normal person, the protein is localized to the nuclear membrane. In your patient, however, the skeletal and cardiac muscle cells do not seem to contain the protein. In neurons, kidney tubular cells, liver cells and spleen cells from a normal person, the protein is not localized to the nucleus but rather it is spread diffusely around the cytoplasm.

Speculate on the function of the protein and how the mutation leads to the disease.

Answer 34

First, analyze the mutation:

Codon number:	180	181	182	183	184
Normal person's DNA:	GAC	TGC	CTG	CCA	ACG
Normal person's RNA:	GAC	UGC	CUG	CCA	ACG
Normal person's protein:	Asp	Cys	Leu	Pro	Thr
Your patient's DNA:	GAC	TGC	CAG	CCA	ACG
Your patient's RNA:	GAC	UGC	CAG	CCA	ACG
Your patient's protein:	Asp	Cys	Gln	Pro	Thr

Your patient's CANP3 has glutamine at position 182 instead of a leucine. This is a very conserved region of the protein. In other words, position 182 is a leucine in both human and rat calpains. Replacing a hydrophobic residue with a polar one is likely to be deleterious, although the precise role of that residue is not known. The calpains are intracellular calcium-activated proteolytic enzymes. CANP3 is particularly prevalent in muscle tissue. Since the disease is recessive, then probably the mutation inactivates the enzyme. One can imagine that the enzyme may play a role in signal transduction. Perhaps it helps to degrade muscle protein for energy. After many years, perhaps some toxic by-products of incomplete digestion accumulate and cause the muscle fibers to decay. It is also possible that the enzyme plays a role in regulating transcription by cleaving the Jun and Fos enzymes or the inhibitor of NF-κB.

REFERENCES

Richard, I., Broux, O., Allamand, V., Fougerousse, F., Chiannilkulchai, N., Bourg, N., Brenguier, L., Devaud, C., Pasturaud, P., Roudaut, C., Hillaire, D., Passos-Bueno, M.-R., Zatz, M., Tischfield, J. A., Fardeau, M., Jackson, C. E., Cohen, D., and Beckmann, J. S. Mutations in the proteolytic enzyme calpain 3 cause limb-girdle muscular dystrophy type 2A. *Cell* 81: 27, 1995.

Answer 35

a. The little blobs are nucleosomes. These form when DNA interacts with histones. Clearly the presence of many GCT triplets favors the formation of nucleosomes. If the DNA is in a nucleosome, then transcription is inhibited. Why this leads to disease is not clear. It is possible that the affected protein kinase plays a role in the regulation of muscular contraction or in muscle metabolism. Interference with muscular contraction or metabolism may, over a long period of time, cause accumulation of some kind of toxic by-product or, alternatively, lead to increasing damage to the muscle cell in some other fashion.

b. There are several other diseases (such as Huntington's disease) where large numbers of triplet repeats occur. These may all operate by the same mechanism. A characteristic of some of these diseases is "genetic anticipation," in which each generation has a larger number of triplet repeats at the same site. The larger the number of repeats, the more likely is nucleosome formation, and the more severe the symptoms. This appears to be the case with your patient's mother and grandmother. Why these repeats are prone to this insertion error is not clear.

Your patient has MYOTONIC DYSTROPHY.

REFERENCES

Fu, Y.-H., Pizzutti, A., Fenwick, R. G., King, J., Rajnarayan, S., Dunne, P.., Dubel, J., Nasser, G. A., Ashizawa, T., De Jong, P., Wieringa, B., Korneluk, R., Perryman, M. B., Epstein, H. F., and Caskey, C. T. An unstable triplet repeat in a gene related to myotonic muscular dystrophy. *Science* 255: 1256, 1992.

Wang, Y.-H., Amirhaeri, S., Kang, S., Wells, R. D., and Griffith, J. D. Preferential nucleosome assembly at DNA triplet repeats from the myotonic dystrophy gene. *Science* 265: 669, 1994.

Answer 36

a. First, analyze the mutation:

Codon number:	2	3	4	5	6	7	8	9	10	11
Normal person's DNA:	ATG	GAG	GCC	ATC	AAG	AAA	AAG	ATG	CAG	ATG
Normal person's RNA:	AUG	GAG	GCC	AUC	AAG	AAA	AAG	AUG	CAG	AUG
Normal person's protein:	Met	Glu	Ala	Ilu	Lys	Lys	Lys	Met	Gln	Met
Your patient's DNA:	ATG	GAG	GCC	ATC	AAG	AAA	AAG	AGG	CAG	ATG
Your patient's RNA:	AUG	GAG	GCC	AUC	AAG	AAA	AAG	AGG	CAG	AUG
Your patient's protein:	Met	Glu	Ala	Ilu	Lys	Lys	Lys	Arg	Gln	Met

Your patient has an arginine at position 9 instead of a methionine. This is a highly conserved region of the tropomyosin molecule. It is also highly basic, and addition of an arginine makes it even more basic. Actin binds to tropomyosin in this area. The positive residues are necessary for the binding. It is likely that addition of another positive residue makes the binding of actin tighter. This could disrupt actin's positioning in the thin filaments and lead to formation of other tropomyosin–actin polymers, such as in the rod bodies.

b. Tropomyosin gene expression is quite complex and their products are different depending on how the mRNAs are spliced. Each gene encodes one product in nonmuscle cells and one in muscle cells. α-Tropomyosin 1 is expressed more in fast muscle fibers and in the heart than in slow muscle fibers. Tropomyosin 3 is expressed more in slow type I muscle fibers.

Your patient has NEMALINE MYOPATHY.

REFERENCES

Gunning, P., Gordon, M., Wade, R., Gahlmann, R., Lin, C.-S., Hardeman, E. Differential control of tropomyosin mRNA levels during myogenesis suggests the existence of an isoform competition-autoregulatory compensation control mechanism. *Dev. Biol.* 138: 443, 1990.

Laing, N. G., Wilton, S. D., Akkari, P. A., Dorosz, S., Boundy, K., Kneebone, C., Blumbergs, P., White, S., Watkins, H., Love, D. R., and Haan, E. A mutation in the α tropomyosin gene *TPM3* associated with autosomal dominant nemaline myopathy. *Nature Genetics* 9: 75, 1995.

Shy, G. M., Engel, W. K., Somers, J. E., and Wanko, T. Nemaline myopathy: A new congenital myopathy. *Brain* 86: 793, 1963.

Answer 37

a. The table shows that the isoforms in normal people are distributed normally. Your patient, however, lacks the muscle isoform in his muscles. Apparently, he compensates in his muscles by having elevated amounts of the brain isoform and the Purkinje cell isoform. Actually, the levels of these isoforms in his skeletal muscle are comparable to the levels in the tissues where they are supposed to be high, namely, the cerebral cortex (brain isoform) and the cerebellum (Purkinje cell isoform). Apparently, these isoforms compensate for the lack of the muscle isoform. Hence, he has no skeletal muscle dystrophy.

b. Although you could not perform a cardiac biopsy on your patient, it is reasonable to suppose that his cardiac muscle would overexpress the brain and Purkinje cell isoforms, just as does his skeletal muscle. This is particularly likely in that normal cardiac muscle already expresses more of the brain isoform than does normal skeletal muscle. Obviously, however, such overexpression cannot compensate for the lack of the muscle isoform. Presumably, the missing exon 1 of the muscle isoform must have some particu-

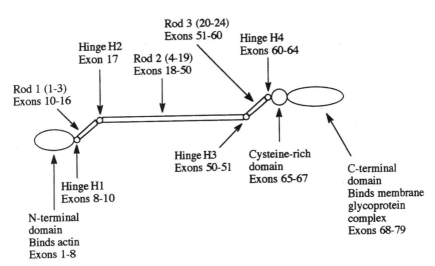

FIGURE A37-1. **Diagram of the dystrophin molecule.** The diagram shows the various domains of the dystrophin molecule. For each domain, the exons in the gene that code for the domain are given. Shown are the N-terminal domain, which interacts with actin, the four hinges, which allow bending of the molecule, the more rigid rod domains, the cysteine-rich domain whose function is not clear, and the C-terminal domain, which is likely to interact with the membrane glycoprotein complex. The dystrophin molecule helps to anchor the actin filaments near the membrane. The rod domains are characterized by repeats of a 109 residue subdomain; there are a total of 24 of these, and these are indicated in parentheses by each rod domain.

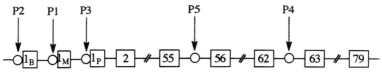

Dystrophin Gene

Promoter:	Exons:	Protein:	Tissues:
P1	1_M, 2-79		Muscle
P2	1_B, 2-79		Brain
P3	1_P, 2-79		Purkinje cells
P4	63-79		Brain, liver, lung, stomach
P5	56-79		Peripheral nerve

○ = Promoter

▢ = Exon

FIGURE A37-2. **Structure of the dystrophin gene and of the various isoforms of dystrophin.** The dystrophin gene and some of its 79 exons are shown at the top. Also indicated as circles are the promoters (P1 to P5). The isoform of dystrophin made in a cell depends in part on which promoter is used. Next to promoters P1 to P3 are different versions of exon 1; thus, these three gene products differ in their N-terminal regions, although the overall domain structures of these three isoforms are almost the same. Activation of the other structures of these three isoforms are almost the same. Activation of the other promoters (P4 and P5) leads to production of highly variant isoforms of dystrophin, whose functions are not at all clear. Still more isoforms are generated by alternative splicing (not shown). In one of these, exon 78 is deleted and the sequence encoded in exon 78 is more hydrophobic; this occurs largely in the fetus. In another, deletion of exon 68 leads to deletion of the whole C-terminal domain. In addition, minor isoforms are generated by deletion of exons 71 to 74, either singly or in various combinations. The functional significance of the isoforms is not clear.

lar function to perform in the heart that is either not necessary in skeletal muscle or that can be performed in skeletal muscle by some other protein not present in cardiac muscle. Hence, he has a cardiac problem.

Your patient has X-LINKED DILATED CARDIOMYOPATHY.

REFERENCES

Muntoni, F., Cau, M., Ganau, A., Congiu, R., Arvedi, G., Mateddu, A., Marrosu, M. G., Cianchetti, C., Realdi, G., Cao, A., and Melis, M. A. Deletion of the dystrophin muscle-promoter region associated with X-linked dilated cardiomyopathy. *N. Engl. J. Med.* 329: 921, 1993.

Muntoni, F., Melis, M. A., Ganau, A., and Dubowitz, V. Transcription of the dystrophin gene in normal tissues and in skeletal muscle of a family with X-linked dilated cardiomyopathy. *Am. J. Hum. Genet.* 56: 151, 1995.

Worton, R. G. and Brooke, M. H. The X-linked muscular dystrophies. C. R. Scriver, A. L. Beaudet, W. S. Sly, and D. Valle (Eds.). *The Metabolic and Molecular Bases of Inherited Disease.* New York: McGraw-Hill, 1995, Vol. III, Chap. 140, p. 4195.

Answer 38

Laminins are important components of the extracellular matrix, specifically of the basal lamina.

First, you need to figure out how the deletion alters the sequence of laminin α2. You will notice that the deletion extends from the third nucleotide in codon 1508 to the first nucleotide in codon 1573.

Normal person:

Codon															
number:	1506	1507	1508	1509	1510	...	1571	1572	1573	1574	1575	1576	1577	1578	1579	1580
DNA:	TGT	GAA	AGG	TGT	GCC	...	TGT	GTT	TTT	TGT	GGA	GAT	GAG	TGC	ACT	GGC
RNA:	UGU	GAA	AGG	UGU	GCC	...	UGU	GUU	UUU	UGU	GGA	GAU	GAG	UGC	ACU	GGC
Protein:	Cys	Glu	Arg	Cys	Ala	...	Cys	Val	Phe	Cys	Gly	Asp	Glu	Cys	Thr	Gly

Your patient:

Codon											
number:	1506	1507	1508	1509	1510	1511	1512	1513	1514	1515	1516
DNA:	TGT	GAA	AGT	TTG	TGG	AGA	TGA	GTG	CAC	TGG	C
RNA:	UGU	GAA	AGU	UUG	UGG	AGA	UGA	GUG	CAC	UGG	C
Protein:	Cys	Glu	Ser	Leu	Trp	Arg	STOP				

Your patient has a massive change in the sequence of laminin α2. Not only are the 64 amino acids encoded by the deleted base pairs missing, but the deletion introduces a frame shift that leads after 4 residues to a STOP codon, which deletes the remainder of the protein. Thus, this laminin α2 is lacking the domains that form the coiled coil structure, where it joins with laminins β1 and γ1. It is unlikely that this truncated laminin will be able to form this trimer.

Laminins are important components of the extracellular matrix, specifically of the basal lamina. The laminin complex of which the α2 chain is a part is one that binds to the glycoprotein called α-dystroglycan. In fact, the portion of laminin complex that binds to α-dystroglycan is the C-terminal domain, which is clearly deleted in your patient. α-Dystroglycan is part of a large complex, some of which is embedded in the membrane of the muscle cell; this complex includes various glycoproteins as well as the large protein dystrophin, which is an intracellular protein that binds to actin. The laminin–dystrophin–glycoprotein connection in essence ties the actin cytoskeleton of the sarcomere to the extracellular matrix and is necessary for the proper function and survival of the muscle cell. Disruptions in the various proteins in this complex give rise to different forms of muscular dystrophy. In the case of your patient, the nonfunctional laminin α2 causes misalignment of the sarcomere components and results ultimately in muscular degeneration.

Your patient has FUKUYAMA CONGENITAL MUSCULAR DYSTROPHY. Laminin α2 is also called merosin, hence, the disease is sometimes referred to as MEROSIN-DEFICIENT CONGENITAL MUSCULAR DYSTROPHY.

REFERENCES

Banker, B. Q. The congenital muscular dystrophies. A. G. Engel and C. Franzini-Armstrong (Eds.). *Myology, Basic and Clinical.* New York: McGraw-Hill, 1994, Vol. 2, Chap. 48, p. 1275.

Ervasti, J. M., and Campbell, K. P. Membrane organization of the dystrophin-glycoprotein complex. *Cell* 66: 1121, 1991.

Gee, S. H., Blacher, R. W., Douville, P. J., Provost, P. R., Yurchenco, P. D., and Carbonetto, S. Laminin-binding protein 120 from brain is closely related to the dystrophin-associated glycoprotein, dystroglycan, and binds with high affinity to the major heparin binding domain of laminin. *J. Biol. Chem.* 268: 14972, 1993.

Helbling-Leclerc, A., Zhang, X., Topaloglu, H., Cruaud, C., Tesson, F., Weissenbach, J., Tomé, F. M. S., Schwartz, K., Fardeae, M., Tryggvason, K. and Guicheney, P. Mutations in the laminin α2-chain gene (*LAMA2*) cause merosin-deficient congenital muscular dystrophy. *Nat. Genet.* 11: 216, 1995.

Tomé, F. M., Evangelista, T., Leclerc, A., Sunada, Y., Manole, E., Estournet, B., Barois, A., Campbell, K. P., and Fardeau, M. Congenital muscular dystrophy with merosin deficiency. *Comptes Rend. Acad. Sci.,* Ser. I, 317: 351, 1994.

Answer 39

First, analyze the mutation:

Codon number:	224	225	226	227	228
Normal person:					
DNA:	CCG	CTC	TGG	GGC	CAG
RNA:	CCG	CUC	UGG	GGC	CAG
Protein:	Pro	Leu	Trp	Gly	Gln
Your patient:					
DNA:	CCG	CTC	TAG	GGC	CAG
RNA:	CCG	CUC	UAG	GGC	CAG
Protein:	Pro	Leu	STOP		

Your patient has a nonsense mutation at codon 226, leading to elimination of the last 29 residues in this protein. The protein is named *emerin*. The C-terminal domain has a hydrophobic domain (residues 224 to 243) thought to be important for anchoring the protein in a membrane. The data from the immunohistochemical experiments shows that, in normal muscle cells, emerin is localized to the nuclear membrane. In your patient, emerin is not located in the nuclear membrane and does not even appear to be present. It appears then that the defect in the emerin molecule prevents it from localizing to the nuclear membrane. The fact that emerin is not present in your patient's muscles suggests that it is rapidly degraded. It is hard to tell what emerin's function is. Perhaps it helps to maintain the architecture of the nuclear membrane or perhaps it helps to anchor the chromosomes to the membrane. If it is absent, it is likely that the nuclei would function poorly. In the course of time, this would lead to degradation of the muscle cells and to the disease.

Why isn't a disease such as this even more serious than it is? It appears that, although nonmuscle cells make emerin, they are not particular about localizing it to the nucleus. Thus, one could speculate that there is a muscle-specific protein that somehow guides or attaches emerin to the nuclear membrane in muscle cells. Perhaps emerin may have another function in other cells, one that does not require it to be in the nucleus.

Your patient has EMERY-DREIFUSS MUSCULAR DYSTROPHY.

REFERENCES

Bione, S., Maestrini, E., Rivella, S., Mancini, M., Regis, S., Romeo, G., and Toniolo, D. Identification of a novel X-linked gene responsible for Emery-Dreifuss muscular dystrophy. *Nat. Genet.* 8: 323, 1994.

Nagano, A., Koga, R., Ogawa, M., Kurano, Y., Kawada, J., Okada, R., Hayashi, Y. K., Tsukahara, T., and Arahata, K. Emerin deficiency at the nuclear membrane in patients with Emery-Dreifuss muscular dystrophy. *Nat. Genet.* 12: 254, 1996.

Worton, R. G. and Brooke, M. H. The X-linked muscular dystrophies. C. R. Scriver, A. L. Beaudet, W. S. Sly, and D. Valle (Eds.). *The Metabolic and Molecular Bases of Inherited Disease.* New York: McGraw-Hill, 1995, Vol. III, Chap. 140, p. 4195.

CHAPTER 11

Skin and Hair

Problem 40

Your patient has skin cancer on her scalp. She has been an avid sunbather for the last 30 years. Biopsy of the tumor shows a somatic mutation in her p53 gene.

a. What are the functions of p53 and how could a mutation in p53 lead to skin cancer?

b. Why might a series of exposures to bright sunlight several days apart be worse than a single long exposure?

Problem 41

Your patient has thickening of the skin on his palms and soles. The thickened areas are surrounded by apparently inflamed margins. You find an alteration in the gene coding for keratin 9. The change is as follows:

Codon number:	156	157	158	159	160	161	162	163
Normal person	ATG	CAG	GAA	CTC	AAT	TCT	CGG	CTG
Your patient:	ATG	CAG	GAA	CTC	TAT	TCT	CGG	CTG

Describe how this change could lead to a skin problem. Include in your analysis a description of how the mutation fits into the structure of keratin.

Problem 42

Your patient has brittle hair, deficient in sulfur. His skin is very rough and he is retarded. You find that he has an altered protein. You purify the protein and add it to a sample of chemically damaged DNA and to another sample of normal DNA. You then add radioactive deoxynucleotides and DNA polymerase and ligase. You find that the incorporation of radioactivity into the two DNA molecules is the same. In contrast, you find that, when you use the equivalent protein from a normal individual in this system, you get considerably more incorporation of radioactivity into the chemically damaged DNA then into the normal DNA. Further research shows that your patient's protein is defective in DNA repair, but your patient is not particularly sensitive to sunlight. Speculate on how the mutation may lead to the symptoms.

Problem 43

Your patient is a 2-week-old infant with widespread blistering and very fragile skin; he has many lesions on his skin. He is suffering from sepsis and his prognosis is poor. You observe a mutation in the sequence of the γ2 subunit of kalinin. The mutation is shown here:

Codon number	92	93	94	95	96	97	98
Normal person:	CTT	AGT	GCT	CGA	TGT	GAC	AAC
Your patient:	CTT	AGT	GCT	TGA	TGT	GAC	AAC

Speculate on how the mutation could lead to loss of kalinin function and on how that could cause the disease.

Problem 44

Your patient was born wrapped in a translucent collodion membrane that dried and cracked shortly afterward. She then developed large brown scales over much of her skin. The skin on her face is so taut that her lips and eyelids are partly everted. You have identified an altered gene in your patient. The sequence of the gene is shown here:

Codon number:	140	141	142	143	144
Normal person:	GTG	CGC	CGC	GGG	CAG
Your patient:	GTG	CGC	CAC	GGG	CAG

a. Describe how the mutation could lead to the disease. Base your argument on the likely three-dimensional structure of the protein.

b. What is the defective protein? What is its function?

Use the following partial protein sequences as a clue to help guide your thinking (these are of factor XIII and related proteins from cows and chickens, and also of your patient's protein):

Your patient's protein (124–146):	NRR EHHTDEYEYDELIXXXXXPF
Human factor XIII (60–82):	NKVDHHTDKYENNKLIVRRGQSF
Bovine protein (17–39):	NGRDHHTADLCRERLVVRRGQPF
Chicken protein (26–48):	NGREHRTEEMGSQQLVVRRGPQF

(The X's are for you to determine).

The three-dimensional structure of factor XIII has been determined. Arginine 78 appears to form a hydrogen bond with the carbonyl oxygen of glycine 253 and to make an electrostatic bond with aspartic acid 191.

Problem 45

Your patient has very thick nails and thickening of the skin on his palms, soles, and tongue. You have sequenced his gene for keratin 6a and found the following:

Codon number:	164	165	166	167	168	169	170	171	172	173	174	175
Normal person	GAA	CAG	ATC	AAG	ACC	CTC	AAC	AAC	AAG	TTT	GCC	TCC
Your patient:	GAA	CAG	ATC	AAG	ACC	CTC	AAC	AAG	TTT	GCC	TCC	TTC

How does the mutation cause the observed symptoms?

Problem 46

Your patient is a man with very thick nails and thickening of the skin of his tongue and mouth. You find the following alteration in the gene coding for his keratin 17:

Codon number:	86	87	88	89	90	91	92	93	94	95
Normal person's DNA:	GCC	ACC	ATG	CAG	AAC	CTC	AAT	GAC	CGC	CTG
Your patient's DNA:	GCC	ACC	ATG	CAG	AAC	CTC	GAT	GAC	CGC	CTG

How might the mutation lead to the observed symptoms?

Problem 47

Your patient has very rough skin with a few patches where the outer layer of skin has fallen away, giving him an appearance of molting. You find an alteration in the gene for his keratin 2e:

Codon number:	115	116	117	118	119
Normal person's DNA:	GAG	GGC	GAG	GAG	TGC
Your patient's DNA:	GAG	GGC	AAG	GAG	TGC

How might the mutation lead to the observed symptoms?

Problem 48

Your patient has patches of white skin on his forehead, chest, and abdomen, as well as on his arms. He has an alteration in one of his genes for the steel factor receptor. The alteration is shown here:

Codon number:	555	556	557	558	559
Normal person:	GTA	CAG	TGG	AAG	GTT
Your patient:	GTA	CAG	TAG	AAG	GTT

He is a heterozygote. His other steel factor receptor gene is normal.

How might this mutation cause the observed symptoms?

Problem 49

You are a dermatologist. Your patient has pronounced blisters on the skin of his hands, elbows, feet, and knees. The hair on his head started falling out when he was 20. Some of his fingernails and all of his toenails are missing. A biopsy sample shows that the dermis and the epidermis of your patient are poorly attached and that the blisters form between the two layers. Electron microscopy of these samples shows poorly formed hemidesmosomes in your patient. One of your other patients recently expired after suffering from a much more severe form of the disease. Your late patient's serum reacts very strongly with an antigen in the dermis–epidermis junction of a normal person but not at all with that of the patient you are now studying; in fact, in the normal person's skin, the binding was localized to the plasma membranes of the hemidesmosomes.

Using appropriate primers you purify and sequence the gene of the antigen from a normal person and from your patient. The partial sequences are shown here:

Codon number:

1250	1260	1268

Normal person:

GGC CCT CCA GGA CCT CCT GGT CCC CCA GGG CCT CGA GGG CCC CCG GGT GTC TCA GGA

Your patient:

GGC CCT CCA GGA CCT CCT GGT CCC CCA GGG CCT TGA GGG CCC CCG GGT GTC TCA GGA

You construct a cDNA probe and measure mRNA levels in your patient's and a normal person's keratinocytes. You find very little mRNA in your patient's keratinocytes compared with the normal person's.

a. What is the function of the hemidesmosome and what are its components?

b. What is the altered protein in your patient?

c. Speculate on how the mutation may lead to the disease.

d. Speculate on the cause of the disease in the patient who died.

Answer 40

a. p53 plays two roles in cells. First, it is apparently induced by UV irradiation and causes a UV-damaged cell to arrest in G1. This arrest allows the cells DNA repair enzymes to fix the damage caused by UV light to their DNA. The second function is to induce apoptosis in response to UV irradiation. Thus, a UV-damaged cell may die. The peeling skin that characterizes sunburn consists of these apoptotic cells. If there is a mutation in p53, induced by UV light, then the mutated cell will not arrest in G1 and any further damage may go uncorrected. Also, the mutated cell is unlikely to undergo apoptosis. Thus, the damaged cells will be able to replicate further. If they have other cancer-causing mutations, they could develop into a malignancy.

b. UV light acts as a selector. Once the original exposure causes a mutation in p53, further exposure will gradually get rid of cells that have normal p53 because they will undergo apoptosis. UV light will thus select for those cells that lack functional p53. Those are precisely the cells that have the greatest likelihood for becoming cancerous.

Your patient has SQUAMOUS CELL CARCINOMA.

REFERENCES

Kamb, A. Sun protection factor p53. *Nature* 372: 730, 1994.

Ziegler, A., Jonason, A. S., Leffell, D. J., Simon, J. A., Sharma, S. W., Kimmelman, J., Remington, L., Jacks, T., and Brash, D. E. Sunburn and p53 in the onset of skin cancer. *Nature* 372: 773, 1994.

Answer 41

First analyze the mutation:

Codon number:	156	157	158	159	160	161	162	163
Normal person's DNA:	ATG	CAG	GAA	CTC	AAT	TCT	CGG	CTG
Normal person's RNA:	AUG	CAG	GAA	CUC	AAU	UCU	CGG	CUG
Normal person's protein:	Met	Gln	Glu	Leu	Asn	Ser	Arg	Leu
Your patient's DNA:	ATG	CAG	GAA	CTC	TAT	TCT	CGG	CTG
Your patient's RNA:	AUG	CAG	GAA	CUC	UAU	UCU	CGG	CUG
Your patient's protein:	Met	Gln	Glu	Leu	Tyr	Ser	Arg	Leu

Your patient has a tyrosine at position 160 instead of an asparagine. This is a highly conserved residue in most intermediate filament proteins, so that fact alone should tell us that any mutation is likely to be deleterious. This position is in the rod domain, which is called a coiled coil. A characteristic of this type of sequence is the heptad repeat *abcdefg* where *a* and *d* are hydrophobic residues that can interact with other hydrophobic residues on another keratin molecule, and *e* and *g* are polar residues that can form hydrogen or ionic bonds with other residues. These links stabilize the heterodimer, which is the fundamental subunit of keratin filaments. Keratin 9 is a type I keratin that can only dimerize with a type II keratin.

The sequence that has been mutated contains the following heptad repeat:

a	*b*	*c*	*d*	*e*	*f*	*g*	*a*
Met	Gln	Glu	Leu	Asn	Ser	Arg	Leu

Replacement of the polar asparagine at the *e* position by a hydrophobic tyrosine would clearly interfere with heterodimer formation. Improper keratin filament formation would cause skin problems.

Your patient has EPIDERMOLYTIC PALMOPLANTAR KERATODERMA.

REFERENCES

Reis, A., Hennies, H.-C., Langbein, L., Digweed, M., Mischke, D., Drechsler, M., Schröck, E., Royer-Pokora, B., Franke, W. W., Sperling, K., and Küster, W. Keratin 9 gene mutations in epidermolytic palmoplantar keratoderma (EPPK). *Nat. Genet.* 6: 174, 1994.

Torchard, D., Blanchet-Bardon, C., Serova, O., Langbein, L., Narod, S., Janin, N., Goguel, A. F., Bernheim, A., Franke, W. W., Lenoir, G. M., and Feunteun, J. Epidermolytic palmoplantar keratoderma cosegregates with a keratin 9 mutation in a pedigree with breast and ovarian cancer. *Nat. Genet.* 6: 106, 1994.

Answer 42

Your patient is defective in a DNA repair enzyme, a DNA helicase. The classic example of a disease caused by a defective DNA repair enzyme is xeroderma pigmentosum. Individuals with that disease must stay out of sunlight because otherwise the sun's ultraviolet radiation may cause them to have skin cancer, due to the lack of the DNA repair enzyme that excises DNA damaged by ultraviolet radiation. However, your patient is not sensitive to sunlight. You have to ask if there is another function for this protein. There probably is. The repair enzyme may also be a component of a transcription initiation complex. If it is defective, inappropriate transcription of certain genes could lead to a developmental problem that could conceivably lead to the observed symptoms.

An interesting question is why your patient's enzyme may be inactive *in vitro* but yet your patient does not seem sensitive to sunlight. The DNA repair enzyme affected by this disease functions *in vivo* as part of a complex, called the "repairosome." It is possible that the repairosome may contain another factor *in vivo* that can compensate for or mask the defect in the DNA repair enzyme. *In vitro*, when the protein is purified away from this hypothetical factor, it will be unable to repair DNA. In individuals with xeroderma pigmentosum, by this model, the DNA repair enzyme is damaged in such a way that the hypothetical factor can neither mask nor compensate for the defect.

Your patient has TRICHOTHIODYSTROPHY.

REFERENCES

Broughton, B. C., Steingrimsdottir, H., Weber, C. A., and Lehmann, A. R. Mutations in the xeroderma pigmentosum group D DNA repair/transcription gene in patients with trichothiodystrophy. *Nat. Genet.* 7: 189, 1994.

Answer 43

The mutation is analyzed as follows:

Codon number:	92	93	94	95	96	97	98
Normal person's DNA:	CTT	AGT	GCT	CGA	TGT	GAC	AAC
Normal person's RNA:	CUU	AGU	GCU	CGA	UGU	GAC	AAC
Normal person's protein:	Leu	Ser	Ala	Arg	Cys		
Your patient's DNA:	CTT	AGT	GCT	TGA	TGT	GAC	AAC
Your patient's RNA:	CUU	AGU	GCU	UGA	UGU	GAC	AAC
Your patient's protein:	Leu	Ser	Ala	STOP			

Your patient has a severely truncated protein. Normally, the γ2 subunit of kalinin contains 1193 amino acids. The mutated form will have 94 amino acids. The γ2 subunit joins with the α3 and β3 subunits to form kalinin, which is a component of the lamina in certain epidermal tissues. Kalinin is very similar to laminin. Kalinin and laminin together may stabilize the basement membrane at the cutaneous dermo-epidermal junction. Loss of kalinin would cause great weakness in this junction and make the skin very fagile, leading to the observed symptoms.

Your patient has HERLITZ'S JUNCTIONAL EPIDERMOLYSIS BULLOSA.

REFERENCES

Aberdam, D., Galliano, M.-F., Vailly, J., Pulkkinen, L., Bonifas, J., Christiano, A. M., Tryggvason, K., Uitto, J., Epstein, E. H., Ortonne, J.-P., and Meneguzzi, G. Herlitz's junctional epidermolysis bullosa is linked to mutations in the gene (LAMC2) for the γ2 subunit of nicein/kalinin (LAMININ-5). *Nat. Genet.* 6: 299, 1994.

Kallunki, P., Sainio, K., Eddy, R., Byers, M., Kallunki, T., Sariola, H., Beck, K., Shows, T. B., and Tryggvason, K. A truncated laminin chain homologous to the

B2 chain: Structure, spatial expression, and chromosomal assignment. *J. Cell Biol.* 119: 679, 1992.

Pulkkinen, L., Christiano, A. M., Airenne, T., Haakana, H., Tryggvason, K., and Uitto, J. Mutations in the γ2 chain gene (LAMC2) of kalinin/laminin 5 in the junctional forms of epidermolysis bullosa. *Nat. Genet.* 6: 293, 1994.

Answer 44

a. The mutation is analyzed as follows:

Codon number:	140	141	142	143	144
Normal person's DNA:	GTG	CGC	CGC	GGG	CAG
Normal person's RNA:	GUG	CGC	CGC	GGG	CAG
Normal person's protein:	Val	Arg	Arg	Gly	Gln
Your patient's DNA:	GTG	CGC	CAC	GGG	CAG
Your patient's RNA:	GUG	CGC	CAC	GGG	CAG
Your patient's protein:	Val	Arg	His	Gly	Gln

In your patient's protein, the arginine at position 142 has been replaced by a histidine. It is clear from the table that your patient's protein is related to factor XIII. Factor XIII, which is a blood coagulation protein, is a transglutaminase. So is your patient's protein, *transglutaminase K*, also known as transglutaminase 1.

Arginine 78 in factor XIII is in the analogous position in the sequence to arginine 142 in transglutaminase 1. It is unlikely that histidine 142 in your patient would be able to form the same bonds. The fact that the arginine at this position is highly conserved supports this hypothesis. In factor XIII, arginine 78 is in the so-called β-sandwich domain, which has no activity, and aspartic 191 and glycine 253 are in the core domain, which has the catalytic activity. It is likely that the interactions between the two domains are critical for the conformational state of the active site. The alteration in the active site is likely to lead to a loss of transglutaminase activity. Thus, proteins that should become cross-linked will not be cross-linked.

b. The mutation apparently inhibits enzyme activity. Transglutaminase K catalyzes the following reactions (Fig. A44-1):

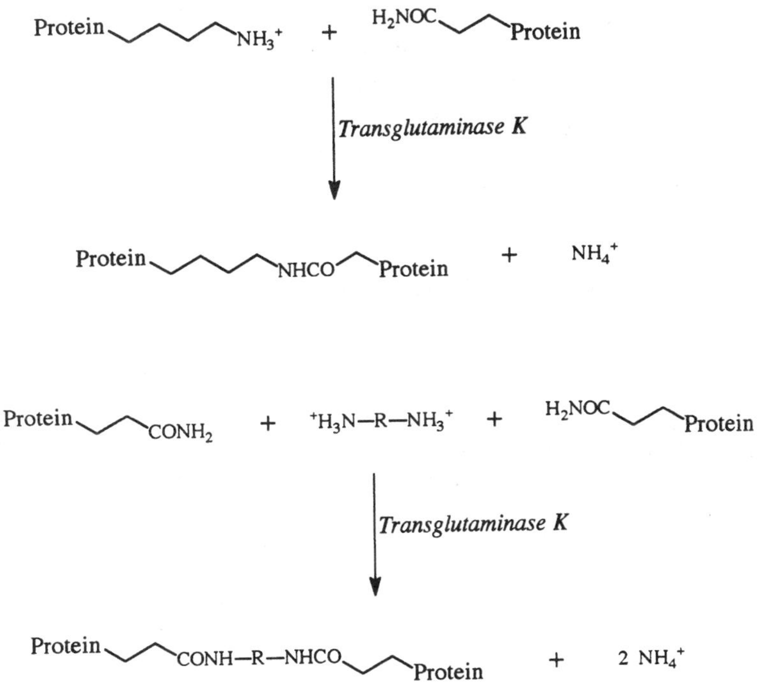

FIGURE A44-1. **Transglutaminase K reaction.** Transglutaminase K makes covalent bonds between protein molecules, either by crosslinking lysine to glutamine residues (top) or by crosslinking glutamines to each other via a polyamine bridge.

1. Protein-lysine + glutamine-protein → protein (glutamyllysine)protein

2. Protein-gln + polyamine + gln-protein → protein (pseudoisopeptide) protein

The polyamine could be putrescine, spermidine, or spermine.

Transglutaminase K plays a critical role in the crosslinking of proteins in the skin, its substrates probably being involucrin, cystatin-α and elafin. Once these proteins are crosslinked, other structural proteins, such as loricrin and keratin can attach to them. If transglutaminase is inhibited, then there will be major skin problems.

The formation of the skin envelope is thought to involve the following steps. First, transglutaminase K crosslinks various substrates to each other and to a 195-kD protein anchored in the membrane. Then transglutaminase E, a different protein, crosslinks loricrin and other proteins to these to form a hard envelope. Then the plasma membrane disappears and is replaced by fatty acids and ceramides, which are covalently attached to the protein envelope.

Your patient has LAMELLAR ICHTHYOSIS.

REFERENCES

Reichert, U., Michel, S., and Schmidt, R. The cornified envelope: A key structure of terminally differentiating keratinocytes. D. Darmon, and M. Blumenberg, Eds. *Molecular Biology of the Skin.* San Diego: Academic Press, 1993, pp. 107–150.

Russell, L. J., DiGiovanna, J. J., Rogers, G. R., Steinert, P. M., Hashem, N., Compton, J. G., and Bale, S. J. Mutations in the gene for transglutaminase 1 in autosomal recessive lamellar ichthyosis. *Nat. Genet.* 9: 279, 1995.

Answer 45

First, analyze the mutation:

Codon number:	164	165	166	167	168	169	170	171	172	173	174	175
Normal person's DNA:	GAA	CAG	ATC	AAG	ACC	CTC	AAC	AAC	AAG	TTT	GCC	TCC
Normal person's RNA:	GAA	CAG	AUC	AAG	ACC	CUC	AAC	AAC	AAG	UUU	GCC	UCC
Normal person's protein:	Glu	Gln	Ilu	Lys	Thr	Leu	Asn	Asn	Lys	Phe	Ala	Ser
Your patient's DNA:	GAA	CAG	ATC	AAG	ACC	CTC	AAC	AAG	TTT	GCC	TCC	TTC
Your patient's RNA:	GAA	CAG	AUC	AAG	ACC	CUC	AAC	AAG	UUU	GCC	UCC	UUC
Your patient's protein:	Glu	Gln	Ilu	Lys	Thr	Leu	Asn	Lys	Phe	Ala	Ser	Phe

Your patient's keratin 6a has a deletion of an entire codon at either position 170 or 171. We cannot tell which because the two codons are identical and consecutive. In either case, we have a deletion of one asparagine. The deletion is near the beginning of the α-helical domain 1A (which starts at position 163). In the structure of keratin, as of any intermediate filament, the α-helical rod domains are the sites where two molecules interact with each other to form the heterodimer. For this to happen, there has to be a heptad repeat (*abcdefg*), where *a* and *d* are hydrophobic residues that can interact with other hydrophobic residues on another keratin molecule, and *e* and *g* are polar residues that can form hydrogen or ionic bonds with other residues. Removing one residue throws the heptad repeats out of phase and may impede the interaction with the other keratin molecule. It is likely that the mutated keratin 6a will be unable to form stable filaments. Since keratin is a major part of the skin, your patient will have skin problems. Since keratin 6a is found in nails, palms, soles, and tongue, it is not surprising that the symptoms are limited to these areas. In the nails, for example, the disorganization of the keratin filaments in the nail bed may make those cells very sensitive to any physical trauma, which might then cause the nail to grow abnormally.

Your patient has PACHYONICHIA CONGENITA, JADAS-SOHN–LEWANDOWSKY FORM.

REFERENCES

Bowden, P. E., Haley, J. L., Kansky, A., Rothnagel, J. A., Jones, D. O., and Turner, R. J. Mutation of a type II keratin gene (K6a) in pachyonychia congenita. *Nat. Genet.* 10: 363, 1995.

Answer 46

The mutation is analyzed as follows:

Codon number:	86	87	88	89	90	91	92	93	94	95
Normal person's DNA:	GCC	ACC	ATG	CAG	AAC	CTC	AAT	GAC	CGC	CTG
Normal person's RNA:	GCC	ACC	AUG	CAG	AAC	CUC	AAU	GAC	CGC	CUG
Normal person's protein:	Ala	Thr	Met	Gln	Asn	Leu	Asn	Asp	Arg	Leu
Your patient's DNA:	GCC	ACC	ATG	CAG	AAC	CTC	GAT	GAC	CGC	CTG
Your patient's RNA:	GCC	ACC	AUG	CAG	AAC	CUC	GAU	GAC	CGC	CUG
Your patient's protein:	Ala	Thr	Met	Gln	Asn	Leu	Asp	Asp	Arg	Leu

Your patient has an aspartic acid at position 92 instead of the normal asparagine. Although this may seem like a small change, aspartic acid is charged, while asparagine is neutral. Also, this position is the 8th position in the α-helical rod domain 1A of keratin 17. This is very close to where the rod domain begins. The asparagine at this position is highly conserved. It is probable that a mutation at this position may interfere with formation of the heterodimer. An analogy may be a lesion at the initiation point of a zipper. A problem here prevents the entire structure from zipping. Conceivably the heterodimer association begins at this spot. A keratin filament containing the mutation may be unable to form stable filaments and thus skin formation would be abnormal. Since keratin 17 is particularly abundant in the nails and the skin of the tongue and mouth, the symptoms appear to be predictably restricted to these areas.

Your patient has PACHYONICHIA CONGENITA, JACKSON–LAWLER FORM.

REFERENCES

McLean, W. H. I., Rugg, E. L., Lunny, D. P., Morley, S. M., Lane, E. B., Swensson, O., Dopping-Hepenstal, P. J. C., Griffiths, W. A. D., Eady, R. A. J., Higgins, C., Navsaria, H. A., Leigh, I. M., Strachan, T., Kunkeler, L., and Munro, C. S. Keratin 16 and keratin 17 mutations cause pachyonychia congenita. *Nat. Genet.* 9: 273, 1995.

Answer 47

The mutation is analyzed as follows:

Codon number:	115	116	117	118	119
Normal person's DNA:	GAG	GGC	GAG	GAG	TGC
Normal person's RNA:	GAG	GGC	GAG	GAG	UGC
Normal person's protein:	Glu	Gly	Glu	Glu	Cys
Your patient's DNA:	GAG	GGC	AAG	GAG	TGC
Your patient's RNA:	GAG	GGC	AAG	GAG	UGC
Your patient's protein:	Glu	Gly	Lys	Glu	Cys

The glutamic acid at position 504 has been replaced by a lysine. This occurs at the very end of the α-helical 2B domain in keratin 2e (the domain ends at residue 508). Normally, the sequence in the rod domains of intermediate filaments is a series of heptads (*abcdefg*) where *a* and *d* are hydrophobic residues that can interact with other hydrophobic residues on another keratin molecule, and *e* and *g* are polar residues that can form hydrogen or ionic bonds with other residues. In this particular heptad (501 to 507), position *d* is occupied by glutamic acid which is not hydrophobic. However, this heptad is at the end of the α-helix and that glutamic acid is highly conserved. Normally, the heptads are interpreted to have the distribution of hydrophobic and polar amino acids that they have so that they can form a heterodimer with another keratin molecule. However, it is possible, in this case, that this very conserved residue at the end of the coiled coil may be involved in linking to other heterodimers, rather than within the heterodimer. If so, replacing this glutamic acid with a positively charged lysine would be very deleterious. If filament formation is abnormal, skin formation will also be abnormal, leading to the observed symptoms.

Your patient has ICHTHYOSIS BULLOSA OF SIEMENS.

REFERENCES

Rothnagel, J. A., Traupe, H., Wojcik, S., Huber, M., Hohl, D., Pittelkow, M. R., Saeki, H., Ishibashi, Y., and Roop, D. R. Mutations in the rod domain of keratin 2e in patients with ichthyosis bullosa of Siemens. *Nat. Genet.* 7: 485, 1994.

Answer 48

The mutation is analyzed as follows:

Codon number:	555	556	557	558	559
Normal person's DNA:	GTA	CAG	TGG	AAG	GTT
Normal person's RNA:	GUA	CAG	UGG	AAG	GUU
Normal person's protein:	Val	Gln	Trp	Lys	Val
Your patient's DNA:	GTA	CAG	TAG	AAG	GTT
Your patient's RNA:	GUA	CAG	UAG	AAG	GUU
Your patient's protein:	Val	Gln	STOP		

Your patient has a termination codon at position 557 instead of a tryptophan. The entire tyrosine kinase portion of this protein is therefore deleted in the mutant.

Steel factor is also known as mast cell growth factor and stem cell factor. Its receptor is called KIT and it is a proto-oncogene. Presumably, a normal KIT factor is required for melanoblast differentiation during embryonic development. Without the tyrosine kinase activity, KIT can bind the steel factor but the cell will not respond, thus inhibiting the growth of melanoblasts. Since the patient is heterozygous for this problem, he will have some normal cells and some areas of normal pigmentation, hence, the patchiness of his condition.

Your patient has PIEBALDISM.

REFERENCES

Ezoe, K., Holmes, S. A., Ho, L., Bennett, C. P., Bolognia, J. L., Brueton, L., Burn, J., Falabella, R., Gatto, E. M., Ishii, N., Moss, C., Pittelkow, M. R., Thompson, E., Ward, K. A., and Spritz, R. A. Novel mutations and deletions of the *KIT* (steel factor receptor) gene in human piebaldism. *Am. J. Hum. Genet.* 56: 58, 1995.

Answer 49

a. Hemidesmosomes are small organelles on the cell membrane that are attached both to the keratin filaments and to laminin. They thus anchor the cytoskeleton of the cell to the basement membrane. The hemidesmosomes contain at least three types of proteins: the 230-kD bullous pemphigoid antigen, the 180-kD bullous pemphigoid antigen, and the integrin $\alpha6\beta4$.

b. First, look at the protein sequence:

Codon number:
```
      1250                                  1260                                  1268
Normal person:
DNA:   GGC CCT CCA GGA CCT CCT GGT CCC CCA GGG CCT CGA GGG CCC CCG GGT GTC TCA GGA
RNA:   GGC CCU CCA GGA CCU CCU GGU CCC CCA GGG CCU CGA GGG CCC CCG GGU GUC UCA GGA
Protein: Gly Pro Pro Gly Pro Pro Gly Pro Pro Gly Pro Arg Gly Pro Pro Gly Val Ser Gly
Your patient:
DNA:   GGC CCT CCA GGA CCT CCT GGT CCC CCA GGG CCT TGA GGG CCC CCG GGT GTC TCA GGA
RNA:   GGC CCU CCA GGA CCU CCU GGU CCC CCA GGG CCU UGA GGG CCC CCG GGU GUC UCA GGA
Protein: Gly Pro Pro Gly Pro Pro Gly Pro Pro Gly Pro STOP
```

You will notice that the protein has a glycine at every third position and is also rich in proline. This is a mark of collagen. Of the three hemidesmosome proteins, only one, the 180-kD bullous pemphigoid antigen, is collagen-like. Thus, this must be the protein that is altered in your patient. In reality, this protein contains many noncollagenous domains. Out of 1433 amino acids, 880 are in noncollagenous domains and 553 are in collagenous domains. The protein has been renamed type XVII collagen. One of the noncollagenous regions contains transmembrane segments. It thus appears that the protein is anchored in the cell membrane. The collagenous domains are thought to be involved in interactions with proteins of the extracellular matrix.

c. The mutation changes an arginine to a STOP codon. This would result in an altered protein lacking its C-terminal region. Although this could be enough to be deleterious, the observation that your patient lacks mRNA for the protein suggests that the mutated mRNA is less stable. This would also explain the fact that the antibody to the protein is unable to find it. Without proper functioning of the hemidesmosomes, the dermis and the epidermis would lose their connection, since the epidermal cells would not be anchored to the basement membrane. This would cause the blistering that you observe.

d. The patient who died clearly had an autoimmune disease; he had an antibody against the same protein that is defective in your living patient. This autoimmune disease is called bullous pemphigoid.

Your patient has GENERALIZED ATROPHIC BENIGN EPIDERMOLYSIS BULLOSA.

REFERENCES

Giudice, G. J., Squiquera, H. L., Elias, P. M., and Diaz, L. A. Identification of two collagen domains within the bullous pemphigoid autoantigen, BP180. *J. Clin. Invest.* 87: 734, 1991.

Giudice, G. J., Emery, D. J., and Diaz, L. A., Cloning and primary structural analysis of the bullous pemphigoid autoantigen BP180. *J. Invest. Dermatol.* 99: 243, 1992.

Hintner, H., and Wolff, K. Generalized atrophic benign epidermolysis bullosa. *Arch. Dermatol.* 118: 365, 1982.

Ishiko, A., Shimizu, H., Kikuchi, A., Ebihara, T., Hashimoto, T., and Nishikawa, T. Human autoantibodies against the 230-kD bullous pemphigoid antigen (BPAG1) bind only to the intracellular domain of the hemidesmosome, whereas those against the 180-kD bullous pemphigoid antigen (BPAG2) bind along the plasma membrane of the hemidesmosome in normal and swine skin. *J. Clin. Invest.* 91: 1608, 1993.

Li, K., Tamai, K., Tan, E. M. L., and Uitto, J. Cloning of type XVII collagen. Complementary and genomic DNA sequences of mouse 180-kilodalton bullous pemphigoid antigen (BPAG2) predict an interrupted collagenous domain, a transmembrane segment, and unusual features in the 5'-end of the gene and the 3'-untranslated region of the mRNA. *J. Biol. Chem.* 268: 8825, 1993.

McGrath, J. A., Gatalica, B., Christiano, A. M., Li, K., Owaribe, K., McMillan, J. R., Eady, R. A. J., and Uitto, J. Mutations in the 180-kD bullous pemphigoid antigen (BPAG2), a hemidesmosomal transmembrane collagen (COL17A1), in generalized atrophic benign epidermolysis bullosa. *Nat. Genet.* 11: 83, 1995.

Uitto, J., and Christiano, A. M. Molecular genetics of the cutaneous basement membrane zone. Perspectives on epidermolysis bullosa and other blistering skin diseases. *J. Clin. Invest.* 90: 687, 1992.

CHAPTER 12

Eyes and Ears

Problem 50

Your patient lost his hearing after taking some gentamicin, which you prescribed for an infection. His mother has a similar history. You have drawn some blood, purified the mitochondrial DNA from his leukocytes, and found a mutation in the gene coding for the mitochondrial 12S rRNA. The mutation is as follows:

    Normal person: GAGGAGACAA
    Your patient: GAGGAGGCAA

The substitution is at position 1555.

a. Explain how this mutation leads to deafness. Hint: see the structure of the corresponding rRNA (16S rRNA) from *Escherichia coli*. see how this mutation might affect the rRNA secondary structure.

b. What other antibiotics would you be careful about prescribing for your patient?

Problem 51

One of your patients (patient A) has difficulty seeing in the dark, so that driving at night is impossible for him. Another patient (patient B) is completely blind, due to retinal degeneration. You are able to clone and sequence their opsin genes. You find that patient A has aspartic acid at position 90 instead of glycine and that patient B has methionine at position 296 instead of lysine. Your search of the literature reveals that, in the absence of 11-*cis*-retinal, there is an electrostatic bond in normal opsin between lysine 296 and glutamic acid 113. The literature also shows that 11-*cis*-retinal forms a Schiff base with the ε-amino group of lysine 296. Finally, molecular modeling suggests that glycine 90, glutamic acid 113 and lysine 296 are very close to each other. You express the different opsins (from a normal individual and from your two patients) and measure the effect of light and 11-*cis*-retinal on their ability to activate transducin. Here are the results:

Source of Opsin	Light	11-*cis*-Retinal	Transducin Activity
Normal person	No	No	0.1
	No	Yes	0.2
	Yes	Yes	11.0
Patient A	No	No	2.0
	No	Yes	0.2
	Yes	Yes	11.0
Patient B	No	No	15.0
	No	Yes	15.0
	Yes	Yes	15.0

Explain how the mutations in your two patients lead to their symptoms and why your patients have such different symptoms.

Problem 52

Your patient is deaf. His stapes is fixed. A CT scan indicates that his internal auditory canal is abnormally dilated and that there is a larger than normal opening between the internal auditory canal and the inner ear compartment. When you did surgery to detach the stapes, you noticed a "gusher" of perilymph. You have found a gene with an altered sequence. Here is the sequence:

Codon number:	331	332	333	334	335	336
Normal person:	CAA	AAA	GAG	AAA	AGA	ATG
Your patient:	CAA	AAA	GAG	GAA	AGA	ATG

Position 334 is in α-helix 3 of the homeodomain of this protein. Analysis of the structures of other proteins in this family shows that position 334 makes contact with the DNA backbone in the major groove of the double helix.

Speculate on how this defect may account for the disease.

Problem 53

Your patient is a 42-year-old deaf diabetic woman. Her brother and her mother have the same symptoms as did her maternal grandmother. She has no signs of muscle weakness. You do a muscle biopsy that shows normal mitochondria. However, when you obtain a sample of her mitochondrial DNA you notice that some (but not all) of it is significantly smaller then normal human mitochondrial DNA. Sequencing of the smaller DNA and comparison with the known map of mitochondrial DNA shows that there is a deletion that extends from nucleotide 4398 to nucleotide 14822. Your patient's mitochondrial DNA lacks the following genes: tRNAs for glutamine, methionine, tryptophan, alanine, asparagine, cysteine, tyrosine, serine, aspartic acid, lysine, glycine, arginine, histidine, leucine, and glutamic acid, parts of complex I (ND2, ND3, ND4L, ND4, Nd5, and ND6), complex III (cytochrome *b*), complex IV (COI, COII, and COIII), and the ATPase (6 and 8).

Why does your patient have symptoms and why are they not more severe? In fact, why is your patient living?

Problem 54

Your patient is blind. He started losing his vision when he was 27. He now has much atrophy of his retina, the retinal pigment epithelium, and the choriocapillaris. He has deposits of lipids all through his fundus, particularly along his Bruch's membrane. You have found an altered gene in your patient. The sequence of a portion of the gene is shown here:

Codon number:	167	168	169	170
Normal person:	GGC	TAC	TGC	AGC
Your patient:	GGC	TGC	TGC	AGC

You are able to clone and express the gene. You do an assay in which you add a radioactive peptide to a connective tissue preparation and measure the release of radioactive amino acids. You also add either the protein from your patient or the equivalent protein from a normal individual. You find the following results:

Additions	Tissue	Radioactivity Released (arbitrary units)
None	No	0
Your patient's protein	No	0
Normal protein	No	0
None	Yes	100
Your patient's protein	Yes	100
Normal protein	Yes	10

The normal protein contains 12 cysteines, all of which are involved in disulfide bridges.

a. What is the function of the protein that is defective in your patient and how might it cause the observed symptoms?

b. Speculate on how the mutation might affect the structure of the protein.

Problem 55

Your patient has normal visual function except for night blindness. Another unusual finding is a gray-white discoloration of the fundus that disappears in the dark but reappears in the light. Your patient has an abnormal gene sequence of a protein called arrestin. The alteration is shown here:

Codon number:	308	309	310
Normal person:	ACA	AAC	CTT
Your patient:	ACA	ACC	TTG

How could this mutation lead to the disease? Be sure that your answer includes an account of the discoloration.

Problem 56

Your patient has no irises around her eyes. She has relatively poor vision. You find an abnormality in the sequence of her PAX6 gene. The abnormality is shown here (after codon 23, the gaps between codons are omitted):

Codon number: 23
Normal person: GAC TCCACCCGGCAGAAGATTGTAGAGCTA....
Your patient: GAC TCCTGCGGACCTCCACCCGGCAGAAGATTGTAGAGCTA....

Describe how this mutation could lead to the observed symptoms.

Answer 50

a. Your patient's mitochondrial rRNA will have a G instead of an A at position 1555. In normal 12S rRNA, position 1555 is at the base of a stem–loop structure. When the structure of mammalian 12S mitochondrial rRNA is compared to that of *Escherichia coli*, it is apparent that *E. coli* has a longer stem–loop structure at that point. Numerous experiments have indicated that this structure is the site of interaction of aminoglycoside antibiotics. One could postulate that the larger the stem–loop structure the tighter the binding of the antibiotics. A mutation in which G replaces A will allow a base pairing with a C at the other side of the stem–loop structure and will make the structure longer and perhaps increase its affinity for aminoglycoside antibiotics (Fig. A50-1). Since the cochlear cells accumulate these antibiotics, they are particularly vulnerable to the effects of this mutation. In fact, binding of aminoglycoside antibiotics will interfere with proper alignment of the tRNAs on the ribosome, since the tRNA binding sites are 4 to 6 nucleotides away from the base of the stem–loop structure (as deduced by analogy with the *E. coli* rRNA). This will in turn cause errors in the translation of the mitochondrial proteins. This could lead to synthesis of nonfunctional components of the electron transport that, in turn, could lead to cell death.

b. Any aminoglycoside antibiotic would be dangerous. Besides gentamicin, these include streptomycin, kanamycin, and neomycin (Fig. A50-2).

Your patient has FAMILIAL ANTIBIOTIC-INDUCED DEAFNESS.

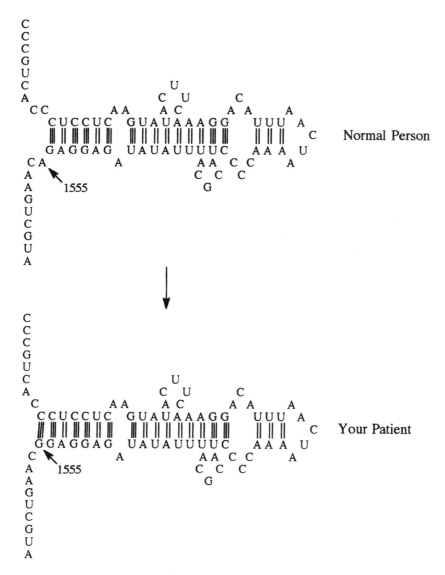

FIGURE A50-1. **Effect of a mutation in your patient's mitochondrial 12S rRNA.**
Notice the stem–loop structure in a normal person (top). The mutation in your patient in which an A is changed to a G at position 1555 allows that G to hydrogen
bond with a C (bottom). The effect is to enlarge the stem–loop structure. It is thought
that increasing the size of this stem–loop structure also increases its ability to bind to
certain antibiotics.

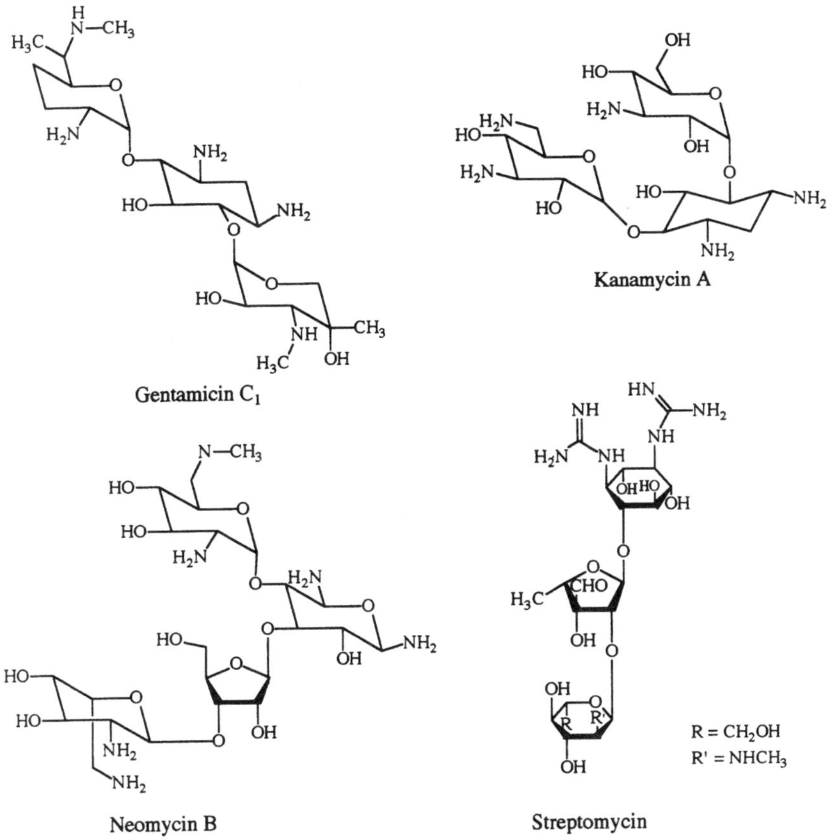

FIGURE A50-2. **Structures of some antibiotics that induce deafness.**

REFERENCES

Prezant, T. R., Agapian, J. V., Bohlmann, M. C., Bu, X., Öztas, S., Qiu, W.-Q., Arnos, K. S. Cortopassi, G. A., Jaber, L., Rotter, J. I., Shohat, M., and Fischel-Ghodsian, N. Mitochondrial ribosomal RNA mutation associated with both antibiotic-induced and non-syndromic deafness. *Nat. Genet.* 4: 289, 1993.

Answer 51

Normal opsin binds to 11-*cis*-retinal at lysine 296. When bound to 11-*cis*-retinal, the protein (now called rhodopsin) is in the "off" con-

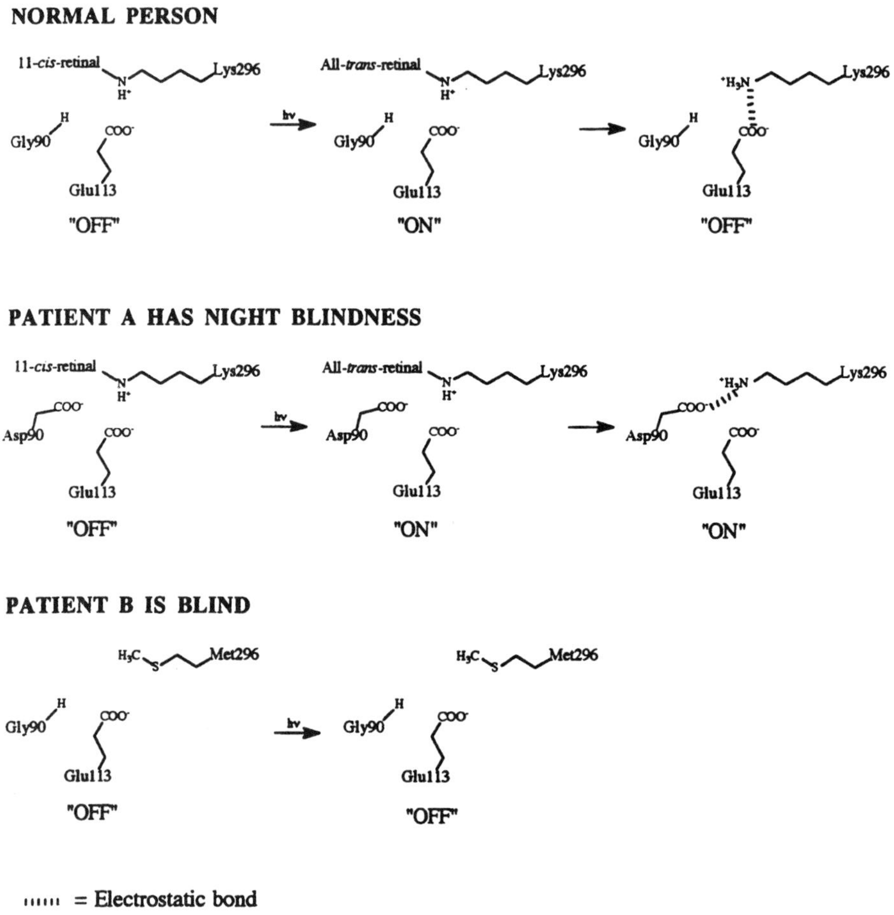

NORMAL PERSON

PATIENT A HAS NIGHT BLINDNESS

PATIENT B IS BLIND

ııııı = Electrostatic bond

FIGURE A51-1. **Structure of the retinal-binding site of the opsin molecule.** The visual pigment retinal binds via a Schiff base to lys296 of opsin. At the point in the visual cycle where the retinal detaches, the ε-amino group of lys296 forms an electrostatic bond with the γ-carboxyl group of glu113 (top); this conformation prevents transduction of the visual signal, so that the protein is OFF. In patient A (middle), the presumably inert gly90 is changed to asp90. When the retinal detaches, the ε-amino group of lys296 is able to form an electrostatic bond with the β-carboxyl of asp90. In this conformation, the transduction is not prevented, so that the protein is ON, leading to night blindness. In patient B (bottom), lys296 is replaced by met296, which cannot bind to retinal, so the opsin molecule is nonfunctional and the patient is blind.

formation. When a photon strikes the chromophore, isomerizing it to all-*trans*-retinal, the protein undergoes a conformational change in which it releases the chromophore. For a moment, the protein is in its "on" conformation in which it activates the transducin. While it is not bound to the retinal, the lysine 296 enters into an electrostatic bond with glutamic acid 113; this bond also keeps the protein in the off conformation. Patient B can obviously not bind to 11-*cis*-retinal since he has a methionine at position 296 and methionine cannot form a Schiff base linkage. Hence patient B is blind. However, since he lacks lysine 296, he cannot form the electrostatic bond with glutamic acid 113, hence his opsin remains in the on position and continues to activate transducin. Having the protein in the on position continuously will lead to retinal degeneration.

Patient A's mutation has a more subtle effect. He has lysine 296, hence, his opsin binds to 11-*cis*-retinal normally and responds normally when light strikes it. However, in the absence of 11-*cis*-retinal, the aspartic acid at position 90 may form an electrostatic bond with lysine 296. Thus, aspartic acid 90 competes with glutamic acid 113 to form this electrostatic bond. However, the electrostatic bond between aspartic acid 90 and lysine 296 does not put the protein into its off conformation. Under normal circumstances, almost all the opsin molecules in the retinal rod cell are bound to 11-*cis*-retinal. However, there are a few hundred in each cell that are not, simply because the normal concentration of 11-*cis*-retinal does not fully saturate the opsin molecules. In these molecules, the lysine 296 will form an electrostatic bond with aspartic acid 90 and the protein will be in the on conformation, thereby sending out a signal. In a situation where the light is very dim (i.e., at night), the signals from such light as there is will be swamped by the background due to the molecules of opsin, which are in the on conformation as a result of this mutation.

Patient A has CONGENITAL NIGHT BLINDNESS and Patient B has RETINITIS PIGMENTOSA.

REFERENCES

Rao, V. R., Cohen, G. B., and Oprian, D. D. Rhodopsin mutation G90D and a molecular mechanism for congenital night blindness. *Nature* 367: 639, 1994.

Answer 52

The mutation is analyzed as follows:

Codon number:	331	332	333	334	335	336
Normal person's DNA:	CAA	AAA	GAG	AAA	AGA	ATG
Normal person's RNA:	CAA	AAA	GAG	AAA	AGA	AUG
Normal person's protein:	Gln	Lys	Glu	Lys	Arg	Met
Your patient's DNA:	CAA	AAA	GAG	GAA	AGA	ATG
Your patient's RNA:	CAA	AAA	GAG	GAA	AGA	AUG
Your patient's protein:	Gln	Lys	Glu	Glu	Arg	Met

Your patient has a glutamic acid at position 334 where a normal individual would have a lysine. This is a drastic change, going from a positive to a negatively charged residue. This is particularly deleterious in this protein because presumably the lysine helps the protein line up on DNA by linking to the negative phosphates. Replacing the lysine with a negatively charged residue may make it impossible for this protein to bind. Clearly, from the description, this protein is a transcription factor. In fact, it is called POU3F4. In your patient this protein is likely to be inactive, in which case certain proteins will not be transcribed. It is likely that this is an auditory system-specific transcription factor. Precisely what proteins have their syntheses affected is not known.

Your patient has X-LINKED MIXED DEAFNESS.

REFERENCES

De Kok, Y. J. M., van der Maarel, S. M., Bitner-Glindicz, M., Huber, I., Monaco, A. P., Malcolm, S., Pembrey, M. E., Ropers, H.-H., and Cremers, F. P. M. Association between X-linked mixed deafness and mutations in the POU domain gene POU3F4. Science 267: 685, 1995.

Answer 53

The disease is clearly maternally inherited, as are mitochondria. Your patient is living because she has some normal mitochondria. The reason that abnormal mitochondria survive is that their DNA is smaller and can reproduce faster. Not given in the list is that the deleted region includes O_L, one of the two origins of mitochondrial DNA replication. It still retains O_H, the other origin. Without O_L, it probably does not replicate as quickly as it would if it still retained O_L. Hence, it is not able to overwhelm the normal muscle mitochondria to cause weakness, but it can affect other tissues to bring on the symptoms that you do see. Why it should be these particular symptoms is unclear.

Your patient has **MATERNALLY TRANSMITTED DIABETES AND DEAFNESS.**

REFERENCES

Ballinger, S. W., Shoffner, J. M., Hedaya, E. V., Trounce, I., Polak, M. A., Koontz, D. A., and Wallace, D. C. Maternally transmitted diabetes and deafness associated with a 10.4 kb mitochondrial DNA deletion. *Nat. Genet.* 1: 11, 1992.

Answer 54

a. The protein in question clearly must function as an inhibitor of proteolytic enzymes. Connective tissue contains a variety of proteolytic enzymes, which are largely metalloproteinases containing zinc ion at their active site. These include at least four types of collagenase, three forms of stromelysin, and matrilysin. The substrates of these metalloproteinases include various forms of collagen, as well as fibronectin, laminin, and proteoglycans. In order to regulate the process, connective tissue also contains inhibitors of these enzymes; these include α_2-macroglobulin and TIMP-1, TIMP-2, TIMP-3, and TIMP-4. In your patient's case, the defective protein is called *TIMP3* (tissue inhibitor of metalloproteinases-3). Overactive metalloproteinases may in time cause destruction of the basal membrane in the retinal region. Why the disease is confined to this area may simply be that the specific inhibitor or metalloproteinase is located in this area.

b. The mutation is analyzed as follows:

Codon number:	167	168	169	170
Normal person's DNA:	GGC	TAC	TGC	AGC
Normal person's RNA:	GGC	UAC	UGC	AGC
Normal person's protein:	Gly	Tyr	Cys	Ser

Your patient's DNA:	GGC TGC TGC AGC
Your patient's RNA:	GGC UGC UGC AGC
Your patient's protein:	Gly Cys Cys Ser

Your patient's protein has a cysteine at position 168 where the normal protein has a tyrosine. This is potentially a very drastic mutation, particularly for a protein that functions extracellularly. The environment is more oxidizing outside the cell. Hence, proteins with cysteines form disulfides. Indeed, the normal protein contains 12 cysteines, each of which is involved in a disulfide. Thus, one of the disulfides involves cys169. The creation of an extra cysteine at position 168 can lead to any of several outcomes. Cysteine 168 could replace cysteine 169 in a disulfide, leaving cysteine 169 free to form other disulfides. Alternatively, cysteine 168 could retain the free sulfhydryl. In the former case, there could be a complete re-arrangement of the structure of the protein. In either case, there is an extra sulfhydryl in the protein; this extra sulfhydryl could react to form a disulfide bridge with a free sulfhydryl in another molecule of the mutated protein or in any other protein. No matter which of these scenarios occurs, it is likely that the protein's conformation or activity will change considerably.

Your patient has SORSBY'S FUNDUS DYSTROPHY.

REFERENCES

Docherty, A. J. P., O'Connell, J., Crabbe, T., Angal, S., and Murphy, G. The matrix metalloproteinases and their natural inhibitors: prospects for treating degenerative tissue diseases. *Trends Biotech.* 10: 200, 1992.

Weber, B. H. F., Vogt, G., Pruett, R. C., Stöhr, H., Felbor, U. Mutations in the tissue inhibitor of metalloproteinases-3 (TIMP3) in patients with Sorsby's fundus dystrophy. *Nat. Genet.* 8: 352, 1994.

Answer 55

The mutation is analyzed as follows:

Codon number:	308	309	310
Normal person's DNA:	ACA	AAC	CTT
Normal person's RNA:	ACA	AAC	CUU
Normal person's protein:	Thr	Asn	Leu

Your patient's DNA:	ACA	ACC	TTG
Your patient's RNA:	ACA	ACC	UUG
Your patient's protein:	Thr	Thr	Leu

Your patient's arrestin has a deletion of a single nucleotide at position 309, causing a frame shift which in turn creates a termination codon. This mutated arrestin lacks 96 amino acids at the C-terminus.

The function of arrestin is to regulate phototransduction. Arrestin competes with transducin for binding to activated rhodopsin (Fig. A55-1). The region 373 to 393 in arrestin is similar to that of a portion of α-transducin. This region is lost in your patient's arrestin. Thus, your patient's arrestin is nonfunctional. With a nonfunctional arrestin, the phototransduction pathway will last a little bit longer. In the dark, your patient's rod cells will be hypersensitive to light and, adapting to that condition, will be unable to react to very faint light. In the presence of normal light, however, the retina will function well, except that the cation channels that are closed as part of the phototransduction process will stay closed longer and the excess cations, such as K^+, will accumulate in the extracellular space, thus causing the discoloration. In the dark, the channels will open and the cations will flow back into the retinal rod cells.

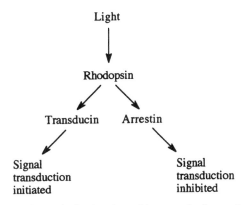

FIGURE A55-1. **Interaction of rhodopsin with transducin and arrestin.** After rhodopsin gets activated by a photon of light, it can bind either to transducin or to arrestin. If it binds to transducin, signal transduction occurs; if it binds to arrestin, then signal transduction is inhibited.

Your patient has OGUCHI DISEASE.

REFERENCES

Fuchs, S., Nakazawa, M., Maw, M., Tamai, M., Oguchi, Y., and Gal, A. A homozygous 1-base pair deletion in the arrestin gene is a frequent cause of Oguchi disease in Japanese. *Nat. Genet.* 10: 360, 1995.

Answer 56

First line up the nucleotides to see what occurred:

Codon number:	23		
Normal person:	GAC	TCC	ACCCGGCAGAAGATTGTAGAGCTA....
Your patient:	GAC	TCCTGCGGACCTCCACCCGGCAGAAGATTGTAGAGCTA....		

Apparently your patient has an insertion of 11 bp in her PAX gene. Since 11 is not divisible by 3, we have a frame shift as a result of this insertion. The effect of this mutation is analyzed as follows:

Codon number:	23	24	25	26	27	28	29	30	31	32	33	34	35
Normal person's DNA:	GAC	TCC	ACC	CGG	CAG	AAG	ATT	GTA	GAG	CTA			
Normal person's RNA:	GAC	UCC	ACC	CGG	CAG	AAG	AUU	GUA	GAG	CUA			
Normal person's protein:	Asp	Ser	Thr	Arg	Gln	Lys	Ilu	Val	Glu	Leu			
Your patient's DNA:	GAC	TCC	TGC	GGA	CCT	CCA	CCC	GGC	AGA	AGA	TTG	TAG	AGC TA.
Your patient's RNA:	GAC	UCC	UGC	GGA	CCU	CCA	CCC	GGC	AGA	AGA	UUG	UAG	AGC UA.
Your patient's protein:	Asp	Ser	Cys	Gly	Pro	Pro	Pro	Gly	Arg	Arg	Leu	STOP	

The result of the frame shift is the introduction of a termination codon at position 35. This will produce a totally nonfunctional PAX6 gene product. Normally, the protein encoded by PAX6 has both paired box and homeobox motifs. These are proteins that can activate transcription. If PAX6 is inactive, certain genes will not get transcribed; among these clearly are the genes coding for the components involved in the development of the iris.

Your patient has ANIRIDIA.

REFERENCES

Martha, A., Ferrell, R. E., Mintz-Hittner, H., Lyons, L. A., and Saunders, G. F. Paired box mutations in familial and sporadic aniridia predicts truncated aniridia proteins. *Am J. Hum. Genet.* 54: 801, 1994.

CHAPTER 13

The Kidney

Problem 57

Your patient has highly impaired kidney function. Biopsy shows that his kidneys have cysts filled with fluid in them. Also, the basement membrane appears to be disorganized. It is difficult to tell which end of the cells is which. Your patient has an abnormality in a gene. The abnormality results in a deletion of the C-terminal region of a protein.

The normal protein is huge (4716 amino acids). When you compare the sequence of this protein to the sequences of other proteins in the data bank, you fail to find any single protein that closely resembles that which is altered in your patient. However, you find that your patient's protein has segments in the sequence that resemble other known proteins. For example, in the N-terminal two-thirds of the protein are numerous potential *N*-glycosylation sites. Also in this region are a lectin domain and four fibronectin-III-related domains. Near the C-terminus are some possible tyrosine kinase sites.

a. Speculate on the role of this protein and how the mutation may lead to disease.

b. How would you treat this patient? Why?

Problem 58

Your patient's kidneys are gradually getting worse. He has repeated episodes of kidney stones. His urinary calcium levels are consistently elevated and there are signs of calcification in his kidneys. You have cloned some of his DNA and found an altered gene in your patient. The partial DNA sequence of the gene is shown here, compared with that for a normal individual:

Codon number:
183 184 185 186 187 188 189 190 191 192 193 194 195 196 197 198 199 200 201 202 203

Normal person:
AGG GGC TAT TTG GGT AAG TGG ACT CTG GTT ATC AAA ACC ATC ACC TTG GTG CTG GCA GTG TCG

Your patient:
AGG GGC TAT TTG GGT AAG TGG ACT CTG GTT ATC AAA ACC ATC ACC TTG GTG CGG GCA GTG TCG

Codon number:
204 205 206 207

Normal person:
TCT GGC TTG AGC

Your patient:
TCT GGC TTG AGC

You did an experiment in which you cloned your patient's gene and expressed it in a *Xenopus* oocyte. You also cloned and expressed the gene from a normal individual in a *Xenopus* oocyte. You then applied a voltage and measured the current across the oocyte membrane in response to the voltage. As another control, you used a *Xenopus* egg that had no exogenous genes expressed. You observed that the ion being transported was chloride. Here are the results:

Gene Expressed in the *Xenopus* Egg	Current (μA)
Normal gene	3.71 ± 0.51
Your patient	0.19 ± 0.03
None	0.27 ± 0.03

In taking the family history of the disease, you observe that your patient's children have no symptoms. However, one of his mother's two brothers has kidney stones, as do three of the six male children of his mother's mother's two sisters. Your patient's uncle with kidney stones actually died of renal failure. On her mother's side, your patient's mother has only one female cousin and this person has no symptoms. When you include some of these people in your study, you find that your patient's mother, although she does not have kidney stones, has elevated urinary calcium levels as do her maternal grandmother, both of her maternal aunts, and the daughter of one these aunts. Not surprisingly, your patient's male relatives who have kidney stones also have elevated calcium levels.

a. How does the mutation cause the disease?

b. Explain the observed distribution of symptoms in your patient's family.

Problem 59

Your patient is a 14-year-old girl with end-stage renal failure. A biopsy at age 7 indicated that her glomerular basement membrane was uneven with unusually thin and unusually thick patches. You find that she has an abnormality in the gene for collagen α4(IV). Here is the sequence of the abnormal gene:

Normal person: GGT TTG CAT GAT GTG GGG CCA CCT GGT CCA GTG GGA
Your patient: GGT TTG CAT GAT GTG GGG CCA CCT AGT CCA GTG GGA

The mutation occurs between interruptions 5 and 6 of the collagenous domain of this protein.

Speculate on how the mutation leads to the disease.

Problem 60

Your patient is a 12-year-old child who suffers from episodes of dehydration. His urine has a very low solute concentration. He drinks about five times more water to satisfy his thirst than does a normal individual. During one of his dehydration episodes, you draw some blood and determine that the plasma concentration of vasopressin is 2 pM. At that time his urinary osmolality is 80 mOsm/kg. A normal individual with that plasma concentration of vasopressin would have a urinary osmolality of 900 to 1300 mOsm/kg.

You find that your patient has an altered gene. The sequence of part of this gene is shown here:

Codon number:	244	245	246	247	248
Normal person:	CCT	GGG	GGG	CGC	CGC
Your patient:	CCT	GGG	GGC	GCC	GCA

The normal protein is 371 amino acids long, whereas your patient's is only 269 residues in length.

a. What is the defective protein likely to be?

b. How might the mutation give rise to the disease?

Problem 61

Your patient has hypertension, which appears to run in her family. Her hypertension does not respond to spironolactone but responds to triamterene. Lowering her salt intake is also helpful. You clone and sequence a gene from your patient and find that it has a mutation, shown here:

Codon number:

| 569 | 570 | 571 | 572 | 573 | 574 | 575 | 576 | 577 | 578 | 579 | 580 | 581 | 582 | 583 | 584 |

Normal person:

AAA GCC AAG GAG TGG TGG GCC TGG AAA CAG GCT CCC CCA TGT CCA GAA

Your patient:

AAA GCC AAG GAG TGG TAG GCC TGG AAA CAG GCT CCC CCA TGT CCA GAA

You express your patient's gene in one set of *Xenopus* oocytes and the normal gene in another set of oocytes. You measure the amiloride-sensitive Na^+ current in across the oocyte membrane. Using antibody to the nonmutated portion of the protein encoded by this gene, you do an immunoprecipitation experiment to measure the total amount of protein expressed by the oocytes. Here are the results:

Source of Gene	Na^+ Current (relative amounts)	Amount of Protein Expressed (relative units)
Normal person	100 ± 3	100
Your patient	210 ± 15	100

In another experiment, you express your patient's gene and a normal gene in a cell line and then, using immunofluorescence and an antibody to the nonmutated portion of the protein, you measure the fluorescence of the cells. Here are the results:

Source of Gene	Fluorescence (relative amounts)	
Normal person	100 ± 1	
Your patient	150 ± 20	$P < 0.025$

a. What is the function of the protein mutated in your patient?

b. How does the mutation cause the disease?

c. Why is your patient insensitive to spironolactone?

Answer 57

a. The mutation is located in the C-terminal area. The description of the protein suggests strongly that it spans the membrane of a cell. First, the lectin domains and the N-glycosylation sites would be extracellular; the tyrosine kinase domain is intracellular. Hence, this protein must be anchored in the membrane. The lectin domain is a region that recognizes oligosaccharide moieties in other proteins. The fibronectin-III-related domains are a characteristic of a large number of cell adhesion proteins. The most likely interpretation, therefore, is that this is a protein involved in cell recognition and adhesion; it is almost certainly required for proper differentiation of the kidney epithelium and for proper organization of the epithelial components, precisely what is missing from your patient. The mutated C-terminus suggests that the intracellular domains of this protein are nonfunctional. This would imply that although the protein is able to recognize and bind to other proteins normally, the cell that expresses this protein is unable to respond properly to this recognition, perhaps by differentiating properly or synthesizing the right matrix components. The protein discussed here has been named *polycystin*. It is encoded by the gene *PKD1*. The disease of your patient is frequent among individuals requiring kidney transplants.

b. A kidney transplant may be a good solution. A new kidney would already be properly formed and differentiated. There would be no reason for your patient's abnormal gene to be expressed.

Your patient has POLYCYSTIC KIDNEY DISEASE.

REFERENCES

Glücksmann-Kuis, M. A., Tayber, O., Woolf, E. A., Bougueleret, L., Deng, N., Alperin, G. D., Iris, F., Hawkins, F., Munro, C., Lakey, N., Duyk, G., Schneider, M. C., Geng, L., Zhang, F., Zhao, Z., Torosian, S., Zhou, J., Reeders, S. T., Bork, P., Pohlschmidt, M., Löhning, C., Kraus, B., Nowicka, U., Leung, A., and Frischauf, A.-M. Polycystic kidney disease: The complete structure of the PKD1 gene and its protein. *Cell* 81: 289, 1995.

Hughes, J., Ward, C. J., Peral, B., Aspinwall, R., Clark, K., San Milláan, J. L., Gamble, V., and Harris, P. C. The polycystic kidney disease 1 (*PKD1*) gene encodes a novel protein with multiple cell recognition domains. *Nat. Genet.* 10: 151, 1995.

Ward, C. J., Peral, B., Hughes, J., Thomas, S., Gamble, V., MacCarthy, A. B., Sloane-Stanley, J., Buckle, V. J., Kearney, L., Higgs, D. R., Ratcliffe, P. J., Harris, P. C., Roelfsema, J. H., Sprult, L., Saris, J. J., Dauwerse, H. G., Peters, D. J. M., Breuning, M. H., Nellist, M., Brook-Carter, P. T., Maheshwar, M. M., Cordeiro, I., Santos, H., Cabral, P., Sampson, J. R., Janssen, B., Hesseling-Janssen, A. L. W., van den Ouweland, A. M. W., Eussen, B., Verhoef, S., Lindhout, D., and Halley, D. J. J. The polycystic kidney disease 1 gene encodes a 14 kb transcript and lies within a duplicated region on chromosome 16. *Cell* 77: 881, 1994.

Answer 58

a. First, you need to look at the effect of the mutation on the protein sequence:

Normal person:

Codon number:

183 184 185 186 187 188 190 191 192 193 194 195 196 197 198 199 200 201 202 203

DNA:

AGG GGC TAT TTG GGT AAG TGG ACT CTG GTT ATC AAA ACC ATC ACC TTG GTG CTG GCA GTG TCG

RNA:

AGG GGC UAU UUG GGU AAG UGG ACU CUG GUU AUC AAA ACC AUC ACC UUG GUG CUG GCA GUG UCG

Protein:

Arg Gly Tyr Leu Gly Lys Trp Thr Leu Val Ilu Lys Thr Ilu Thr Leu Val Leu Ala Val Ser

Codon number:

204 205 206 207

DNA:

TCT GGC TTG AGC

RNA:

UCU GGC UUG AGC

Protein:

Ser Gly Leu Ser

Your patient:

Codon number:

183 184 185 186 187 188 189 190 191 192 193 194 195 196 197 198 199 200 201 202 203

DNA:

AGG GGC TAT TTG GGT AAG TGG ACT CTG GTT ATC AAA ACC ATC ACC TTG GTG CGG GCA GTG TCG

RNA:

AGG GGC UAU UUG GGU AAG UGG ACU CUG GUU AUC AAA ACC AUC ACC UUG GUG CGG GCA GUG UCG

Protein:

Arg Gly Tyr Leu Gly Lys Trp Thr Leu Val Ilu Lys Thr Ilu Thr Leu Val Arg Ala Val Ser

Codon number:

204   205   206   207

DNA:

TCT GGC TTG AGC

RNA:

UCU GGC UUG AGC

Protein:

Ser   Gly   Leu   Ser

Your patient has an arginine at position 200 in this protein where a normal person has a leucine. What is this protein? The experiment in the *Xenopus* egg suggests that it may be a channel protein permitting chloride to pass across the membrane. Your patient's protein is clearly unable to pass any chloride ion, since transport of chloride is not above background level. In fact, it is a chloride channel protein called CLC-5.

Why is the mutation deleterious for the function of the protein? If you look at the sequence of amino acids, you will see that from positions 185 to 202 thirteen out of 18 residues are hydrophobic. On either side of this region, the residues are significantly less hydrophobic. Eighteen residues is about right for a membrane-spanning domain. This is entirely consistent with your protein being a chloride channel protein. Replacing the hydrophobic leucine with an arginine may cause the channel to be oriented inappropriately in the hydrophobic membrane. The result would be an inactive channel, which is apparently what your patient has.

If your patient is unable to reabsorb chloride, it is likely that calcium will also fail to be reabsorbed and will accumulate in the kidney tubules and eventually precipitate, causing kidney stones and calcification of the kidney.

b. The pattern of inheritance of the disease suggests that it is maternally inherited, in that only your patient's male relatives get the kidney stones. The gene is therefore probably on the X chromosome. Some women who are carriers, however, would express both the normal and the defective protein in which case they might have some hypercalciuria, but the calcium levels would not be high enough to cause kidney stones.

Your patient has DENT'S DISEASE (HYPERCALCIURIC NEPHROLITHIASIS).

Interestingly, other mutations in the same gene can cause other similar, but distinct, diseases, namely, X-linked recessive nephrolithiasis, and X-linked recessive hypophosphatemic rickets. It is perhaps significant that kidney stones are over twice as common in men than in women.

REFERENCES

Fisher, S. E., van Bakel, I., Lloyd, S. E., Pearce, S. H. S., Thakker, R. V., and Craig, I. W., Cloning and characterization of CLCN5, the human kidney chloride channel gene implicated in Dent disease (an X-linked hereditary nephrolithiasis). *Genomics* 29: 598, 1995.

Lloyd, W. E., Pearce, S. H. S., Fisher, S. E., Steinmeyer, K., Schwappach, B., Scheinman, S. J., Harding, B., Bolino, A., Devoto, M., Goodyer, P., Rigden, S. P. A., Wrong, O., Jentsch, T. J., Craig, I. W., and Thakker, R. V., A common molecular basis for three inherited kidney stone diseases. *Nature* 379: 445, 1996.

Answer 59

The mutation is analyzed as follows:

Normal person's DNA:	GGT	TTG	CAT	GAT	GTG	GGG	CCA	CCT	GGT	CCA	GTG	GGA
Normal person's RNA:	GGT	UUG	CAU	GAU	GUG	GGG	CCA	CCU	GGU	CCA	GUG	GGA
Normal person's protein:	Gly	Leu	His	Asp	Val	Gly	Pro	Pro	Gly	Pro	Val	Gly
Your patient's DNA:	GGT	TTG	CAT	GAT	GTG	GGG	CCA	CCT	AGT	CCA	GTG	GGA
Your patient's RNA:	GGU	UUG	CAU	GAU	GUG	GGG	CCA	CCU	AGU	CCA	GUG	GGA
Your patient's protein:	Gly	Leu	His	Asp	Val	Gly	Pro	Pro	Ser	Pro	Val	Gly

Your patient has a serine instead of a glycine. In the collagenous domain every third residue is glycine. Clearly, here we have a serine replacing one of those glycines. This in effect adds another interruption to a sequence that contains several interruptions. Type IV collagen, which occurs in basement membranes, is much more flexible than the type I collagen, which forms strong fibers. However, the collagenous segments of type IV collagen are thought to form triple helices with other type IV collagen molecules to form a network of thin fibers, which constitutes the basement membrane. Possibly this mutation disrupts that network and leads to a gradual weakening of the basement membrane and ultimately to renal failure.

Your patient has ALPORT SYNDROME.

REFERENCES

Mochizuki, T., Lemmink, H. H., Mariyama, M., Antignac, C., Gibler, M.-C., Pirson, Y., Verellen-Dumoulin, C., Chan, B., Schröder, C. H., Smeets, H. J., and Reeders, S. T. Identification of mutations in the α3(IV) and α4(IV) collagen genes in autosomal recessive Alport syndrome. *Nat. Genet.* 8: 77, 1994.

Answer 60

a. Your patient is able to make vasopressin (Fig. A60-1), but he does not seem to respond to it. Hence, the defective protein is likely to be the *vasopressin* V_2 receptor, since this is involved with water transport in the kidney. There is also a vasopressin V_1 receptor, but this is involved with vasoconstriction.

b. The mutation is analyzed as follows:

Codon number:	244	245	246	247	248
Normal person's DNA:	CCT	GGG	GGG	CGC	CGC
Normal person's RNA:	CCU	GGG	GGG	CGC	CGC
Normal person's protein:	Pro	Gly	Gly	Arg	Arg
Your patient's DNA:	CCT	GGG	GGC	GCC	GCA
Your patient's RNA:	CCU	GGG	GGC	GCC	GCA
Your patient's protein:	Pro	Gly	Gly	Ala	Ala

Your patient has a deletion of one nucleotide in codon 246; this causes a frame shift that introduces a STOP codon at position 270, leading to a truncated protein.

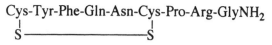

FIGURE A60-1. **Structure of vasopressin.**

Your patient's V_2 receptor is missing a substantial portion of the C-terminal domain. This is the domain that interacts with the G protein leading to cAMP synthesis and to activation of water transport from the renal collecting tubule back into the blood. Without this segment, the transport system is not activated, large amounts of water are excreted and the urine is hypotonic. The most dangerous result of this is dehydration.

Your patient has NEPHROGENIC DIABETES INSIPIDUS.

REFERENCES

Merendino, J. J., Spiegel, A. M., Crawford, J. D., O'Carroll, A.-M., Brownstein, M. J., Lolait, S. J. A mutation in the vasopressin V_2-receptor gene in a kindred with X-linked nephrogenic diabetes insipidus. *New Engl. J. Med.* 328: 1538, 1993.

Rosenthal, W., Seibold, A., Antaramian, A., Lonergan, M., Arthus, M.-F., Hendy, G. N., Birnbaumer, M., and Bichet, D. G. Molecular identification of the gene responsible for congenital nephrogenic diabetes insipidus. *Nature* 359: 233, 1992.

Answer 61

a. The protein is a sodium channel protein. In fact, it is the epithelial Na^+ channel protein, a protein involved in reabsorption of sodium ion from the kidney. This protein consists of three distinct but similar subunits called α, β, and γ. As it happens, the γ subunit is altered in your patient.

b. The mutation is analyzed as follows:

Codon number:	569	570	571	572	573	574	575	576	577	578	579	580	581	582	583	584
Normal person:																
DNA:	AAA	GCC	AAG	GAG	TGG	TGG	GCC	TGG	AAA	CAG	GCT	CCC	CCA	TGT	CCA	GAA
RNA:	AAA	GCC	AAG	GAG	UGG	UGG	GCC	UGG	AAA	CAG	GCU	CCC	CCA	UGU	CCA	GAA
Protein:	Lys	Ala	Lys	Glu	Trp	Trp	Ala	Trp	Lys	Gln	Ala	Pro	Pro	Cys	Pro	Glu

Your patient:
DNA: AAA GCC AAG GAG TGG TAG GCC TGG AAA CAG GCT CCC CCA TGT CCA GAA
RNA: AAA GCC AAG GAG UGG UAG GCC UGG AAA CAG GCU CCC CCA UGU CCA GAA
Protein: Lys Ala Lys Glu Trp STOP

Your patient has a STOP codon at position 574. This means that the C-terminal portion of the protein is deleted. How does this affect the function? Clearly the protein is able to function since your *Xenopus* experiments showed that sodium ion could be transported with the mutant protein. In fact, your patient's protein transports sodium more than twice as much as does the normal protein. Does the *Xenopus* oocyte simply express more of the mutant than of the normal protein? You know that is not true because you measured expression of the normal and mutant proteins and found them to be the same. This would imply that your patient's protein transports sodium better. Is that true? Not necessarily. Your antibody experiment showed that there was considerably more of your patient's protein in the membrane than there was of the normal protein. This suggests that the problem with your patient's protein is one of its localization rather than one of its function.

There is clearly too much of your patient's protein in the membrane. Therefore, either too much gets targeted to the membrane or else not enough gets internalized into the cell. The results of your experiment are consistent with either model. However, the deleted portion of your patient's protein contains the sequence Pro-Pro-Pro-Lys-Tyr-Asn-Thr-Lys (residues 623 to 630). This bears some similarity to a sequence in other membrane proteins that is thought to be required for internalization. If this is a valid comparison, the likelihood is that the deletion prevents the channel from internalizing.

Either way, there is too much channel in the membrane, hence too much Na^+ gets reabsorbed into the blood from the kidney, and hypertension results.

c. Spironolactone is an antagonist of aldosterone, which increases sodium transport.

Your patient has LIDDLE DISEASE.

REFERENCES

Hansson, J. H., Nelson-Williams, C., Suzuki, H., Schild, L., Shimkets, R., Lu, Y., Canessa, C., Iwasaki, T., Rossier, B., and Lifton, R. P. Hypertension caused by a truncated epithelial sodium channel γ subunit: Genetic heterogeneity of Liddle syndrome. *Nat. Genet.* 11: 76, 1995.

Liddle, G. W., Bledsoe, T., and Coppage, W. S. A familial renal disorder simulating primary aldosteronism but with negligible aldosterone secretion. *Trans. Assoc. Am. Phys.* 76: 199, 1963.

Schild, L., Canessa, C. M., Shimkets, R. A., Gautschi, I., Lifton, R. P., and Rossier, B. C. A mutation in the epithelial sodium channel causing Liddle disease increases channel activity in the *Xenopus laevis* oocyte expression system. *Proc. Natl. Acad. Sci. USA* 92: 5699, 1995.

Snyder, P. M., Price, M. P., McDonald, F. J., Adams, C. M., Volk, K. A., Zeiher, B. G., Stokes, J. B., and Welsh, M. J. Mechanism by which Liddle's syndrome mutations increase activity of a human epithelial Na^+ channel. *Cell* 83: 969, 1995.

CHAPTER 14

Bones and Cartilage

Problem 62

Your patient is a 12-year-old boy with a cleft palate and hearing impairment. He has had gradually worsening problems with his joints. His father and his father's brother had similar symptoms, but his brother does not have the symptoms and neither does his mother. His parents are unrelated to each other. You find that he has an alteration in a gene coding for collagen α2(XI). Here is the alteration:

Codon number: 976   977   978   979   980   981
Normal person: GGT CCC CCC GGC CTC CCC gtgagtactgcct
Your patient: GGT CCC CCC GGC CTC CCC atgagtactgcct

(Uppercase letters are in the exons, lowercase in the intron).

Your patient's collagen α2(XI) is 18 residues shorter than that of a normal individual.

Speculate on how the change could lead to the observed symptoms.

Problem 63

Your patient is a 2-year-old boy with a poorly developed nasal cartilage and a cleft palate. X-rays show a stippling in regions of growing bone; the stippling is apparently due to irregularity in calcification. You find that your patient has an altered gene whose sequence is shown here:

Codon number: 136 137 138 139 140 141
Normal person: AAA GGC TAT GCC ACT GGA
Your patient: AAA GTC TAT GCC ACT GGA

You find out that, in a related protein, the residue equivalent to 137 is located at the point where an α-helix meets a β-sheet.

You do the following experiment. You incubate a cell extract with 4-methylumbelliferyl sulfate and measure the release of sulfate. You find that the release of sulfate was about 3% of that which you would expect in cells of a normal individual. Further studies on the normal protein show that it can be inactivated by heating to 50°C and that it is not inhibited by dehydroepiandrosterone sulfate. It is, however, inhibited by warfarin.

a. What protein is defective in your patient?

b. How does the mutation lead to the observed symptoms? Speculate.

c. Another one of your patients is a pregnant woman who takes warfarin for a blood coagulation disorder against your advice. What is likely to happen to her baby?

Problem 64

Your patient is a dwarf with short limbs and a very large head. You do a biopsy and culture some of your patient's chondrocytes. You add fibroblast growth factor to them and find that they do not undergo mitosis in response; in contrast, normal chondrocytes are stimulated to divide by this factor. You find that your patient has an altered protein. Here is a portion of the sequence of this protein (residues 372 to 396), compared to that of a normal individual:

Normal person: VYAGILSYGVGFFLFILVVAAVTLC
Your patient: VYAGILSYRVGFFLFILVVAAVTLC

a. What protein is defective in your patient?

b. How might the defect give rise to the observed symptoms?

Problem 65

Your patient is a 2-month-old girl with premature fusion of the sutures in the skull, causing a cloverleaf-shaped skull. She also has bulging eyes. Some of this condition you are able to correct with surgery. You observe an abnormality in a gene in your patient. The sequence of a part of the gene is shown here:

Codon number: 341   342   343   344   345
Normal person: ACG   TGC   TTG   GCG   GGT
Your patient: ACG   TGC   TTG   GCA   GGT

From a biopsy sample, taken at the time of surgery, you culture some bone cells. You incubate the bone cells with an antibody to phosphotyrosine and measure the antibody binding. Comparing these results to those obtained with cells from a normal individual, you find the following:

Source of Cells	Addition	Phosphotyrosine Level (arbitrary units)
Normal person	None	10
Normal person	Fibroblast growth factor	100
Your patient	None	10
Your patient	Fibroblast growth factor	50

a. What protein is defective in your patient and how is the function affected?

b. How might the mutation explain the results of your experiment and your patient's symptoms?
A helpful piece of information is the sequence of the intron–exon boundary elsewhere in the gene:

tgtgtctgttgtagCACT

Lowercase letters denote the intron and uppercase the exon.

Problem 66

Your patient died of respiratory failure a few minutes after birth. His bones were very poorly formed. You find that he had a mutation in the gene coding for fibroblast growth factor receptor 3. The sequence in the area of the mutation is shown here:

Codon number: 246 247 248 249 250 251 252 253 254 255 256
Normal person: CTG GAG CGC TCC CCG CAC CGG CCC ATC CTG CAG
Your patient: CTG GAG TGC TCC CCG CAC CGG CCC ATC CTG CAG

How might the mutation lead to the symptoms?

Problem 67

Your patient is a 22-year-old man in need of a hip replacement. He is short with short hands and loose joints. He also has scoliosis. He needs a new hip because of degeneration of the cartilage in some of his joints. He has a mutation in the gene encoding cartilage oligomeric matrix protein. The alteration in the sequence is shown here:

Codon number: 367 368 369 370 371 372 373 374 375 376 377
Normal person: CGG GGC GAT GCG TGC GAC GAC GAC ATC GAC GGC
Your patient: CGG GGC GAT GCG TGC GAC GAC ATC GAC GGC GAC

This mutation occurs in the region of the protein, which is a calmodulin-like domain.

You do a biopsy and observe that the rough endoplasmic reticulum of your patient is swollen with some kind of material.

Speculate on how the mutation in the protein could lead to the disease.

Problem 68

Your patient is 7 feet tall and has a variety of physical deformities, including a cleft palate (repaired), a groove in the middle of his tongue, and severe dental malocclusion. You have isolated the gene for a protein called glypican-3 and sequenced it. Your patient has a deletion removing three exons from this gene.

How might a defect in this protein give rise to abnormal growth?

Problem 69

There are several allelic forms of the vitamin D receptor. A study has shown a correlation between the presence of a certain allele and the bone density in an individual. The different alleles differ significantly in their 3'-untranslated regions. In one experiment, the luciferase gene was fused onto the 5' end of the 3'-untranslated regions of each of two of the vitamin D receptor alleles. When the fused gene was transfected into kidney cells in culture, the luciferase activity varied greatly as a function of which allele's 3'-untranslated region was present. How do these results relate to osteoporosis?

Answer 62

Your patient has a mutation in the first nucleotide of his intron. This undoubtedly causes exon skipping, leading to a molecule of collagen α2(XI) that is 18 residues shorter than that of a normal person. Collagen XI is one of the fiber-forming collagens, together with collagen types I, II, III, and V. Collagen XI is associated almost exclusively with cartilage. It forms triple helices that consist of one molecule each of α2(XI), α1(XI), and α1(II) Presumably, the defective collagen α2(XI) could not bind correctly to the other collagen molecules, or, if bound, could not form a larger fiber structure. However, the pattern of inheritance described for your patient suggests that the disease is dominant. Thus, your patient presumably also makes molecules of normal α2(XI). This would suggest that the abnormal protein present in your patient could participate in some of the interactions, in fact, enough to poison further assembly. For example, perhaps your patient's α2(XI) could form a triple helix with the other types of collagen, but those triple helices might not form fibers. In such a case, the presence of the normal α2(XI) might alleviate the symptoms but not eliminate them. The abnormal fiber formation might lead to the joint problems and the other symptoms.

Your patient has STICKLER SYNDROME.

REFERENCES

Kimura, T., Cheah, K. S. E., Chan, S. D. H., Lui, V. C. H., Mattei, M.-G., van der Rest, M., Ono, K., Solomon, E., Ninomiya, Y., and Olsen, B. R. The human α2(XI) collagen (COL11A2) chain. Molecular cloning of cDNA and genomic DNA reveals characteristics of a fibrillar collagen with differences in genomic organization. *J. Biol. Chem.* 264: 13910, 1989.

Vikkula, M., Mariman, E. C. M., Lui, V. C. H., Zhidkova, N. I., Tiller, G. E., Goldring, M. B., van Beersum, S. E. C., de Waal Malefijt, M. C., van den Hoogen, F. H. J., Ropers, H.-H., Mayne, R., Cheah, K. S. E., Olsen, B. R., Warman, M. L., and Brunner, H. G. Autosomal dominant and recessive osteochondriodysplasias associated with the *COL11A2* locus. *Cell* 80: 431, 1995.

Answer 63

a. The defeceive protein is clearly one that removes sulfates from certain substrates. The common sulfatases are inhibited by dehydroepiandrosterone sulfate, but this one is not. The common ones are not heat labile, but this one is. The defective enzyme is thus *arylsulfatase E*, distinct from arylsulfatases A, B, and C.

b. The mutation is analyzed as follows:

Codon number:	136	137	138	139	140	141
Normal person's DNA:	AAA	GGC	TAT	GCC	ACT	GGA
Normal person's RNA:	AAA	GGC	UAU	GCC	ACU	GGA
Normal person's protein:	Lys	Gly	Tyr	Ala	Thr	Gly
Your patient's DNA:	AAA	GTC	TAT	GCC	ACT	GGA
Your patient's RNA:	AAA	GUC	UAU	GCC	ACU	GGA
Your patient's protein:	Lys	Val	Tyr	Ala	Thr	Gly

Your patient has a valine at position 137 instead of a glycine. Glycine is highly conserved at this position in the other arylsulfatases. Glycine is often found at positions where two parts of the structure come together such as an α-helix and a β-sheet. The small side chain of glycine allows the two structures to fit together well. Replacing this glycine with a valine is bound to be deleterious to activity, since it will alter the protein conformation. The actual role of arylsulfatase E in bone and cartilage growth is not known; however, a major component of cartilage are glycosaminoglycans, which are sulfated. In the recycling that accompanies growth, these glycosaminoglycans may be substrates for arylsulfatases. It is reasonable to speculate that arylsulfatase E may participate in this process, even though we don't know exactly what it does.

c. Arylsulfatase E is inhibited by warfarin (Fig. A63-1), which is not the case for the similar arylsulfatase C. You might expect that a pregnant woman who takes warfarin may have a child with the same symptoms as the patient with a defective arylsulfatase E and that is indeed the case. That is called "warfarin embryopathy."

For further information about sulfatases, see Problem 4.

Your patient has X-LINKED RECESSIVE CHONDRODYSPLASIA PUNCTATA.

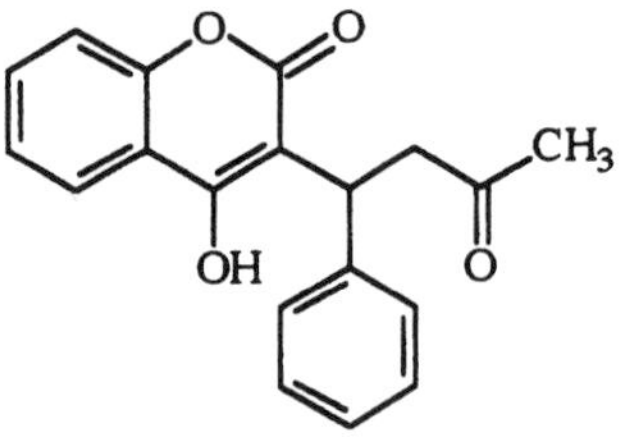

FIGURE A63-1. **Structure of warfarin.**

REFERENCES

Franco, B., Meroni, G., Parenti, G., Levilliers, J., Bernard, L., Gebbia, M., Cox, L., Maroteaux, P., Sheffield, L., Rappold, G .A., Andria, G., Petit, C., and Ballabio, A. A cluster of sulfatase genes on Xp22.3: Mutations in chondrodysplasia punctata (CDPX) and implications for warfarin embryopathy. *Cell* 81: 15, 1995.

Answer 64

a. The defective protein must be a receptor for fibroblast growth factor present in chondrocytes. In fact it is *fibroblast growth factor receptor-3.*

b. Your patient has an arginine at position 380 instead of glycine. As you can see from the sequence, this is a highly hydrophobic region of the protein. It is likely, in fact, to be the transmembrane domain that this type of receptor has to have. Appearance of a charged and bulky amino acid is very likely to disrupt the transmembrane α-helix. In fact, it may make it impossible for the signal to be transduced across the membrane, from the domain that recognizes and binds to fibroblast growth factor to the cytoplasmic domain that contains the tyrosine kinase activity. In short, the receptor would not respond to the fibroblast growth factor. Thus, the cartilage cells would not proliferate and there would be serious problems in forming cartilage.

Your patient has ACHONDROPLASIA.

REFERENCES

Rousseau, F., Bonaventure, J., Legeal-Mallet, L., Pelet, A., Rozet, J.-M., Maroteaux, P., Le Merrer, M., and Munnich, A. Mutations in the gene encoding fibroblast growth factor receptor-3 in achondroplasia. *Nature* 371: 252, 1994.

Answer 65

a. The defective protein is likely to be the receptor for fibroblast growth factor, which has a cytoplasmic tyrosine kinase domain. In fact, it is *fibroblast growth factor receptor 2*. The defect appears to be that it does not respond well to fibroblast growth factor.

b. The mutation is analyzed as follows:

Codon number:	341	342	343	344	345
Normal person's DNA:	ACG	TGC	TTG	GCG	GGT
Normal person's RNA:	ACG	UGC	UUG	GCG	GGU
Normal person's protein:	Thr	Cys	Leu	Ala	Gly
Your patient's DNA:	ACG	TGC	TTG	GCA	GGT
Your patient's RNA:	ACG	UGC	UUG	GCA	GGU
Your patient's protein:	Thr	Cys	Leu	Ala	Gly

You will notice that your patient's mutation involves changing a G to an A in codon 344. Neverthess, the codon still codes for alanine. However, you now have an AG in the nucleotide sequence. Elsewhere in the gene there is an AG at a splice site. Your patient may have formed a splice site in his gene that would then create the following sequence:

DNA:	acgtgcttggcag GTA A
RNA:	GUA A
Protein:	Val

It is possible that some of the proteins made will have a frame shift in this region of the receptor. It is conceivable that this might lead to a low level of activity even in the presence of fibroblast growth factor. This could cause abnormal bone deposition, leading to the premature fusion of the skull.

Your patient has CROUZON SYNDROME.

REFERENCES

Reardon, W., Winter, R. M., Rutland, P., Pulleyn, L. J., Jones, B. M., and Malcolm, S. Mutations in the fibroblast growth factor receptor 2 gene cause Crouzon syndrome. *Nat. Genet.* 8: 98, 1994.

Answer 66

The mutation is analyzed as follows:

Codon number:	246	247	248	249	250	251	252	253	254	255	256
Normal person's DNA:	CTG	GAG	CGC	TCC	CCG	CAC	CGG	CCC	ATC	CTG	CAG
Normal person's RNA:	CUG	GAG	CGC	UCC	CCG	CAC	CGG	CCC	AUC	CUG	CAG
Normal person's protein:	Leu	Glu	Arg	Ser	Pro	His	Arg	Pro	Ilu	Leu	Gln
Your patient's DNA:	CTG	GAG	TGC	TCC	CCG	CAC	CGG	CCC	ATC	CTG	CAG
Your patient's RNA:	CUG	GAG	UGC	UCC	CCG	CAC	CGG	CCC	AUC	CUG	CAG
Your patient's protein:	Leu	Glu	Cys	Ser	Pro	His	Arg	Pro	Ilu	Leu	Gln

Your patient had a cysteine at position 248 instead of an arginine. Position 248 is in the extracellular region of fibroblast growth factor receptor 3. It is located between the second and third immunoglobulin-like domains of the protein. These latter domains are regions that contain disulfide bridges between cysteines. The mutation introduces a new cysteine into the sequence. The effect may be to rearrange the disulfide bridges. The new arrangement may lead to a drastically different conformation, one in which the ligand, fibroblast growth factor, does not bind. In such a case, the effect would be that growth of many tissues would not be stimulated. Fibroblast growth factor receptor 3 is expressed most highly in bone and nervous tissue. The likely effect of this mutation would be to inhibit bone growth, which would be very serious and almost certainly lethal. Nervous system anomalies are difficult to study in infants who live for only a short time, but they have been observed in this syndrome.

Your patient has THANATOPHORIC DYSPLASIA.

REFERENCES

Tavormina, P. L., Shiang, R., Thompson, L. M., Zhu, Y.-Z., Wilkin, D. J., Lachman, R. S., Wilcox, W. R., Rimoin, D. L., Cohn, D. H., and Wasmuth, J. J. Thanatophoric dysplasia (types I and II) caused by distinct mutations in fibroblast growth factor receptor 3. *Nat. Genet.* 9: 321, 1995.

Answer 67

The mutation is analyzed as follows:

Codon number:	367	368	369	370	371	372	373	374	375	376	377
Normal person's DNA:	CGG	GGC	GAT	GCG	TGC	GAC	GAC	GAC	ATC	GAC	GGC
Normal person's RNA:	CGG	GGC	GAU	GCG	UGC	GAC	GAC	GAC	AUC	GAC	GGC
Normal person's protein:	Arg	Gly	Asp	Ala	Cys	Asp	Asp	Asp	Ilu	Asp	Gly
Your patient's DNA:	CGG	GGC	GAT	GCG	TGC	GAC	GAC	ATC	GAC	GGC	GAC
Your patient's RNA:	CGG	GGC	GAU	GCG	UGC	GAC	GAC	AUC	GAC	GGC	GAC
Your patient's protein:	Arg	Gly	Asp	Ala	Cys	Asp	Asp	Ilu	Asp	Gly	Asp

Your patient has a deletion of an entire codon. Instead of three aspartic acids in a row, he has only two.

Cartilage oligomeric matrix protein is an adhesion protein similar to thrombospondin. The protein appears to form links with glycosaminoglycans and with other adhesion proteins. The protein exists as a pentamer of five subunits. The removal of an aspartic acid residue could have a serious effect on your patient's protein for two reasons. First, it is likely, by analogy with calmodulin, that these aspartic acid residues are involved in binding calcium. In this case, the protein may bind less calcium. Although the precise role of calcium in the activity of cartilage oligomeric matrix protein is not known, it is likely that a decrease in calcium binding may alter some of the adhesion interactions, perhaps by changing the conformation. Also, removal of an amino acid from the sequence may move the other amino acids into a different configuration that would also lead to an alteration in the conformation and perhaps in the binding properties of the protein. It is tempting to imagine that the altered protein forms pentamers that cannot be secreted and hence accumulate in the endoplasmic reticulum. This could account for the microscopic observations. This would also imply that a smaller amount of cartilage oligomeric matrix protein would be secreted into the extracellular matrix. Thus, the mutant protein might either interact differently with other proteins or else might not be secreted. Assuming your patient is heterozygous for this condition, there would be many normal subunits of cartilage oligomeric matrix protein. If the pentamers form in the endoplasmic reticulum, then the mutation would result in lesser secretion of normal pentamers as well, since 31/32 of the pentamers would contain at least one abnormal chain.

Your patient has PSEUDOACHONDROPLASIA.

REFERENCES

Briggs, M. D., Hoffman, S. M. G., King, L. M., Olsen, A. S., Mohrenweiser, H., Leroy, J. G., Mortier, G. R., Rimoin, D. L., Lachman, R. S., Gaines, E. S., Cekleniak, J. A., Knowlton, R. G., and Cohn, D. H. Pseudoachondroplasia and multiple epiphyseal dysplasia due to mutations in the cartilage oligomeric matrix protein gene. *Nat. Genet.* 10: 330, 1995.

Answer 68

Glypican-3 is a small proteoglycan that is anchored to the membrane of certain mesodermal cells via a glycosylphosphatidylinositol linkage. The protein binds to insulin-like growth factor 2 (IGF2). It is hypothesized that glypican regulates the interaction of IGF2 with its receptor, perhaps to diminish the reaction in some way. If the glypican-3 is abnormal, it is possible that it may not bind so well to IGF2, and the result would be a potentiation of IGF2 action and hence greater and probably abnormal growth.

Your patient has SIMPSON–GOLABI–BEHMEL SYNDROME.

REFERENCES

Pilia, G., Hughes-Benzie, R. M., MacKenzie, A., Baybayan, P., Chen, E. Y., Huber, R., Neri, G., Cao, A., Forabosco, A., and Schlessinger, D. Mutations in *GPC3*, a glypican gene, cause the Simpson-Golabi-Behmel overgrowth syndrome. *Nat. Genet.* 12: 241, 1996.

Weksberg, R., Squire, J. A., and Templeton, D. M. Glypicans: A growing trend. *Nat. Genet.* 12: 225, 1996.

Answer 69

Apparently, the sequence of the 3'-untranslated region influences the rate of transcription of the gene. Thus, certain alleles will be transcribed more than others. People who have these alleles will have more vitamin D receptors and will therefore have a higher bone density and less of a tendency to osteoporosis.

REFERENCES

Morrison, N. A., Qi, J. C., Tokita, A., Kelly, P. J., Crofts, L., Nguyen, T. V., Sambrook, P. N., and Elsman, J. A. Prediction of bone density from vitamin D receptor alleles. *Nature* 367: 284, 1994.

CHAPTER 15

The Gonads

Problem 70

Your patient is a 5-year-old child who appears to be a girl, although her karyotype shows she is XY. Her kidneys function poorly and her internal genitalia are poorly developed. Your patient has an altered gene, part of whose sequence is shown here:

Normal person: CATACAGGTAAAACAAgtgcgtaaact
Your patient: CATACAGGTAAAACAAgtgcataaact

(Uppercase letters are exons, lowercase denotes introns.)

The gene in question has 4 zinc-finger domains,and the mutation occurs between the third and fourth domains.

You do an experiment in which you construct a minigene containing the area around the mutation. You construct the same minigene from a normal person. You transfect this gene into cultured cells, then after two days purify the RNA, construct cDNAs and measure and sequence the cDNAs. From the normal minigene, you find two cDNAs expressed, one 86 nucleotides long and one 77 nucleotides long. The longer cDNA contains the sequence:

CATACAG<u>GTAAAACAA</u>...

The shorter cDNA contains the sequence:

CATACAG...

It appears to be lacking 9 nucleotides, which are underlined in the sequence of the larger cDNA.

In contrast to the normal minigene, expression of the mutated minigene leads to expression of only the 86 nucleotide cDNA with a sequence identical to that produced from the normal minigene.

a. What is the matter with your patient's gene expression and why does it lead to a problem?

b. Speculate on how this mutation could lead to symptoms.

Problem 71

Your patient is a 20-year-old man with hypospadia, an abnormal opening of the urethra on the underside of the penis. He has a small penis and his testicles have only partly descended into the scrotum. He also developed enlarged breasts at puberty. The levels of testosterone in his plasma are normal. You find that there is a major alteration in the gene for the androgen receptor. The alteration is that about 600 bp of intron 2 are missing. This does not include either splice site or any part of an exon but does include an apparent branch point sequence TATCAAC. You analyze the mRNA for the androgen receptor. You find that there are two mRNAs. About 92% lacks exon 3 entirely, while the remaining 8% is the normal mRNA. The protein encoded by the mutant mRNA is unable to activate transcription.

Explain how this deletion could give rise to the observed phenotype.

Answer 70

a. Your patient has a mutation in the intron to a gene. It appears that under normal circumstances your patient's protein can be expressed in different forms depending on how the splicing occurs. Your patient's mutation has altered the splicing pattern in the gene. Thus, only the longer isoform of the protein is expressed in your patient.

b. If you assume that each isoform of this protein has a job to do, then your patient is compromised because she will lack one of the isoforms. The missing protein is evidently a DNA-binding protein, probably a transcription factor that controls expression of various genes. In fact, the gene is called *WT1* (Wilms tumor 1), and it is normally expressed as four isoforms arising from alternative splicing. If these genes are not transcribed, one could imagine having improper development. In fact, this gene is expressed largely in the genitourinary system.

Your patient has DENYS–DRASH SYNDROME.

REFERENCES

Bruening, W., Bardeesy, N., Silverman, B. L., Cohn, R. A., Machin, G. A., Aronson, A. J., Housman, D., and Pelletier, J. Germline intronic and exonic mutations in the Wilms' tumour gene (*WT1*) affecting urogenital development. *Nat. Genet.* 1: 144, 1992.

Haber, D. A., and Housman, D. E. Wilms tumor. C. R. Scriver, A. L. Beaudet, W. S. Sly, D. Valle, J. B. Stanbury, J. B. Wyngaarden, and D. S. Fredrickson (Eds.). *The Metabolic and Molecular Bases of Inherited Disease.* New York: McGraw-Hill, 1995, Vol. I, Chap. 13, p. 665.

Answer 71

The branch point sequence (TATCAAC) plays an important role in splicing. The third A in this sequence is linked temporarily to the 5' end of the intron. If this branch point sequence is deleted, it is difficult for correct splicing to occur, even if the actual splice sites are still present. However, it appears that there is another sequence in the mutated intron 2 that could serve as a branch point, although not very effectively. Thus, some normally spliced mRNA will be made. The abnormally spliced mRNA encodes an inactive androgen receptor that will not respond to testosterone and dihydrotestosterone. Thus, your patient will not exhibit normal virilization. However, the small amount of normal androgen receptor will respond. Hence, there will be partial development of the secondary sexual characteristics.

Your patient has REIFENSTEIN SYNDROME.

REFERENCES

Griffin, J. E., McPhaul, M. J., Russell, D. W., and WIlson, J. D. The androgen resistance syndromes: Steroid 5α-reductase 2 deficiency, testicular feminization, and related disorders. C. R. Scriver, A. L. Beaudet, W. S. Sly, D. Valle, J. B. Stanbury, J. B. Wyngaarden, and D. S. Fredrickson (Eds.). *The Metabolic and Molecular Bases of Inherited Disease.* New York: McGraw-Hill, 1995, Vol. II, Chap. 95, p. 2967.

Ris-Stalpers, C., Verleun-Mooijman, M. C. T., de Blaeij, T. J. P., Degenhart, H. J., Trapman, J., and Brinkmann, A. O. Differential splicing of human androgen receptor pre-mRNA in X-linked Reifenstein syndrome, because of a deletion involving a putative branch site. *Am. J. Hum. Genet.* 54: 609, 1994.

CHAPTER 16

The Brain and the Nervous System

Problem 72

Your patient is a 55-year-old man who has gradually been losing the use of his limbs. The loss of function started at the periphery and has spread inward gradually. You obtain some of his lymphocytes and do an assay in which you measure the ability to inhibit nitrite formation from hydroxylammonium chloride. You find that this activity is 73% of that of normal. Your patient has an altered gene, shown here:

Codon number:	40	41	42
Normal person:	GAA	GGC	CTG
Your patient:	GAA	AGC	CTG

a. What is the defective gene in your patient?

b. How might the mutation lead to the symptoms?

Problem 73

Your patient has just died of a disease characterized by jerky movements, loss of cognition, and psychiatric disturbances. His father and his maternal grandmother had the same disease. You examine your patient's genome and find an altered gene. Here is a portion of the sequence of the gene for a normal person:

Codon number:

| 15 | 16 | 17 | 18 | 19 | 20 | 21 | 22 | 23 | 24 | 25 | 26 | 27 | 28 | 29 | 30 | 31 | 32 | 33 | 34 | 35 |

DNA:

AAG TCC TTC CAG CAG CAG CAG CAG CAG CAG CAG CAG CAG CAG CAG CAG CAG CAG CAG CAG CAG

Codon number:

| 36 | 37 | 38 | 39 | 40 | 41 | 42 | 43 | 44 | 45 | 46 | 47 | 48 | 49 | 50 |

DNA:

CAG CAG CAG CAG CAG CCG CCA CCG CCG CCG CCG CCG CCG CCG CCT

Your patient has the following sequence inserted between codons 40 and 41:

CAGCAGCAGCAGCAGCAGCAGCAGCAGCAGCAGCAGCAGCAGCAGCAGCA GCAGCAGCAGCAGCAGCAGCAGCAGCAGCAGCAGCAGCAGCAGCAGCAG.

In separate experiments you observe the following:

1. An antibody to the normal protein shows that the protein is located in many different tissues.

2. In neurons, the protein is associated with synaptic vesicles.

3. A peptide consisting of 60 residues of glutamine binds to the enzyme glyceraldehyde-3-phosphate dehydrogenase, whereas a peptide consisting of 20 glutamines does not.

4. You observe that the normal protein binds to another protein, which you call protein X. Protein X is enriched in the brain.

5. Autopsy of your patient shows degeneration of the medium spiny neurons of the caudate putamen.

6. When animals are given drugs that inhibit energy metabolism, they show similar symptoms as your patient and similar degeneration in their brains.

a. Speculate on how the altered protein could cause disease.

b. If the protein is found throughout the body, why are the symptoms mainly neurological?

c. What is significant about long stretches of glutamine?

d. One of your patient's ancestors was hanged as a witch in 1653 in New England. Why is this relevant?

Problem 74

Your patient is a 35-year-old woman who has been growing progressively senile. You have discovered that certain of her cells have an overproduction of a fragment of β-amyloid precursor protein called Aβ. You observe that your patient has an abnormal gene, which is not the gene for the β-amyloid precursor protein. The mutation in your patient leads to her having a glutamic acid at position 246 instead of an alanine. You analyze the sequence of this protein, and your computer tells you that certain areas are likely to correspond to transmembrane segments; these are 82 to 100, 133 to 154, 164 to 183, 195 to 213, 221 to 238, 244 to 262, and 408 to 299. Your search for other proteins with similar sequences has found that the most similar is a protein from the nematode worm *Caenorhabditis elegans*. The nematode protein, called SPE-4, has been studied. It is located in the Golgi apparatus of sperm-forming cells of the nematode. Mutations in this protein interfere with associations with other cellular structures made by the Golgi during meiosis.

Speculate on how the mutation may lead to the disease.

Problem 75

Your patient is mentally retarded and has very broad thumbs and broad big toes. You find that he has an altered gene, whose sequence is shown here:

Codon number: 352   353 354 355 356 357 358 359 360 361 362 363 364 365

Normal person: AAA CTG ATA CAG CAG CAG CTG GTT CTA CTG CTT CAT GCT CAT

Your patient: AAA CTG ATA CAG CAG TAG CTG GTT CTA CTG CTT CAT GCT CAT

The protein encoded by this gene in a normal individual has several interesting properties. First, one of its domains, residues 462 to 661, binds to a transcription factor called CREB, but only when CREB is phosphorylated. The binding of this protein to CREB stimulates the transcription-enhancing properties of CREB.

a. Describe the pathway in which this protein and CREB participate and how it is regulated.

b. Speculate on how the mutation could lead to the observed symptoms.

Problem 76

The immediate cause of Alzheimer's disease appears to be the abnormal deposition in the brain of a peptide called Aβ, which is a fragment of a larger protein called β-amyloid precursor protein. Two proteins that may also be involved are α_1-antichymotrypsin and apolipoprotein E. The first of these, α_1-antichymotrypsin, is synthesized by astrocytes; it is also present in the blood. Apolipoprotein E occurs in various allelic forms, called E2, E3, and E4. The relative amounts of these alleles vary among individuals. In the United States, for example, 1.3% of the population is E2/E2, 58% is E3/E3, 3% is E4/E4, 22% is E2/E3, 2% is E2/E4, and 14% is E3/E4.

You do an experiment in which you measure the ability of various proteins to induce Aβ to polymerize. You measure polymerization by electron microscopy by a technique in which you count the number of crossovers of filaments in a given grid area. Here are the results:

Proteins Added	Filament Crossovers/ Unit Area
α_1-Antichymotrypsin	0
Apolipoprotein E2	0
Apolipoprotein E3	0
Apolipoprotein E4	0
Aβ	15
Aβ + serum albumin	10
Aβ + apolipoprotein A1	20
Aβ + apolipoprotein A2	5
Aβ + α_1-antichymotrypsin	100
Aβ + apolipoprotein E2	35
Aβ + apolipoprotein E3	105
Aβ + apolipoprotein E4	200
Aβ + apolipoprotein E4 + apolipoprotein E2	20

a. Put these facts together into a theory of Alzheimer's disease.

b. Speculate on how you could use the information gained in this experiment to predict which individuals are most likely and least likely to get Alzheimer's disease.

c. Speculate as to the function of the β-amyloid precursor protein in a normal individual.

Problem 77

Your patient has a benign tumor of his Schwann cells. He also has an altered protein.

You do an experiment in which you incubate the protein $p21^{ras}$ with this protein and measure what percentage of the guanine nucleotide bound to the $p21^{ras}$ is GTP. Here are the results:

Protein	GTP/(GTP + GDP) on $p21^{ras}$ (%)
Your patient's protein	50
Normal protein	5

a. What is the role of the protein that appears to be defective in your patient? How could the mutation cause the observed problem?

b. Why might an inhibitor of farnesyltransferase help this disease?

Problem 78

Your patient has a benign tumor of his Schwann cells, confirmed by gadolinium-enhanced MRI. You find that he has an altered gene in his tumor cells, although not in his other cells. The alteration is shown here:

Codon number: 54   55   56   57   58   59   60
Normal person: CTG GGC CTC CGA GAA ACC TGG
Your patient: CTG GGC CTC TGA GAA ACC TGG

The protein encoded by this gene is 597 amino acids long.

You find that the sequence of this protein is very similar to that of ezrin, moesin, and erythrocyte protein 4.1. Based on this finding, speculate on the function of the protein and how the mutation leads to the disease.

Problem 79

Your patient has had a progressive disease for several years. She is now 12 years old. Her symptoms began with weakness of her leg muscles, which made her clumsy when she ran and gave her a strange gait when walking. She has lost a good deal of sensory function in her feet, leading to ulcers at points of pressure. You find an alteration in her gene for connexin 32. The alteration is shown here:

Codon number:	139	140	141	142	143
Normal person:	GTG	GTG	TTC	CGG	CTG
Your patient:	GTG	GTG	TTC	TGG	CTG

Speculate on how the mutation leads to the disease.

Problem 80

Your patient is a girl who was clinically normal until she was 6 years old. Then she began having apparent epileptic seizures, increasing in frequency and intensity until they were happening up to 100 times each day. She is unable to talk or play and is essentially bed ridden. A sample of your patient's blood was fractionated. The immunoglobulin G fraction was able to evoke an electrical potential in some cultured mouse neurons; the currents were abolished by 6-cyano-7-nitroquinoxaline-2,3-dione. In a related experiment, you injected some purified glutamate receptor R3 into a rabbit and the rabbit started having seizures.

a. What is the origin of your patient's disease?

b. How would you treat this patient?

Answer 72

a. The defective gene is *superoxide dismutase 1*. Human tissues contain two groups of isoforms of superoxide dismutase. One group, superoxide dismutase 1, or copper/zinc superoxide dismutase, is found in the cytosol of most cells. Most of the members of this group are dimers of A and B subunits, the specific isoforms arising from different combinations of the subunits. Also in this group is a tetrameric isoform found largely in blood plasma; this isoform is sometimes referred to as extracellular superoxide dismutase. This isoform is thought to scavenge superoxide in the plasma. The second group of isoforms, manganese superoxide dismutase, is less well known; it is found in mitochondria, where it may help to defend against oxidative damage arising during inflammation.

b. The mutation is analyzed as follows:

Codon number:	40	41	42
Normal person's DNA:	GAA	GGC	CTG
Normal person's RNA:	GAA	GGC	CUG
Normal person's protein:	Glu	Gly	Leu
Your patient's DNA:	GAA	AGC	CTG
Your patient's RNA:	GAA	AGC	CUG
Your patient's protein:	Glu	Ser	Leu

Your patient has a serine at position 41 instead of a glycine. This glycine is the first residue of a β-sheet. It is also at the boundary of the active site loop containing copper ion. It is likely that this mutation causes a decrease in activity by altering the conformation of the protein. It is conceivable that the increased superoxide levels may be deleterious to neurons. One could imagine that they might be particularly harmful to structures in cells that last a long time. Such a structure are the neurofilaments that may accu-

$$O_2^- \cdot \; + \; O_2^- \cdot \; + \; 2\,H^+ \; \longrightarrow \; H_2O_2 + O_2$$

FIGURE A72-1. **Superoxide dismutase reaction.**

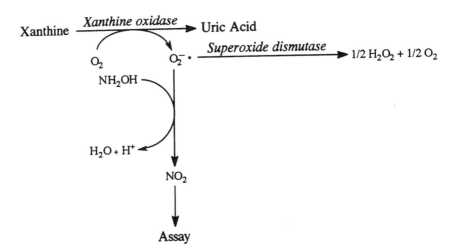

FIGURE A72-2. **Assay for superoxide dismutase activity.** In this assay, $O_2^-\cdot$ is generated by the action of xanthine oxidase on xanthine. The $O_2^-\cdot$ thus generated reacts with NH_2OH to generate NO_2, whose presence can be measured. Superoxide dismutase will react with $O_2^-\cdot$ in a competing reaction and will thus inhibit NO_2 production.

mulate abnormally under these conditions and inhibit axonal transport. This would eventually lead to neuronal cell death. The effect would be most marked at first in the longest neurons, namely, those in the periphery.

Your patient has AMYOTROPHIC LATERAL SCLEROSIS.

REFERENCES

Collard, J.-F., Côté, F. and Julien, J.-P. Defective axonal transport in a transgenic mouse model of amyotrophic lateral sclerosis. *Nature* 375: 61, 1995.

Crapo, J. D., Oury, T., Rabouille, C., Slot, J. W., and Chang, L.-Y. Copper,zinc superoxide dismutase is primarily a cytosolic protein in human cells. *Proc. Natl. Acad. Sci. USA* 89: 10405, 1992.

Elstner, E. F. and Heupel, A. Inhibition of mitrite formation from hydroxylammonium chloride: A simple assay for superoxide dismutase. *Anal. Biochem.* 70: 616, 1976.

Fridovich, I. Superoxide dismutases. *Adv. Enzymol.* 58: 61, 1986.

Pattichis, K., Louca, L. L., and Glover, V. Quantitation of soluble superoxide dis-

mutase in rat striata, based on the inhibition of nitrite formation from hydroxylammonium chloride. *Anal. Biochem.* 221: 428, 1994.

Tsuda, T., Munthasser, S., Fraser, P. E., Percy, M. E., Rainero, I., Vaula, G., Pinessi, L., Bergamini, L., Vignocchi, G., McLachlan, D. R. C., Tatton, W. G., and St. George-Hyslop, P. Analysis of the functional effects of a mutation in *SOD1* associated with familial amyotrophic lateral sclerosis. *Neuron* 13: 727, 1994.

Answer 73

a. First, analyze the nature of the mutation:

Codon number:

15	16	17	18	19	20	21	22	23	24	25	26	27	28	29	30	31	32	33	34	35

DNA:

AAG TCC TTC CAG CAG CAG CAG CAG CAG CAG CAG CAG CAG CAG CAG CAG CAG CAG CAG CAG CAG

RNA:

AAG UCC UUC CAG CAG CAG CAG CAG CAG CAG CAG CAG CAG CAG CAG CAG CAG CAG CAG CAG CAG

Protein:

Lys Ser Phe Gln Gln Gln Gln Gln Gln Gln Gln Gln Gln Gln Gln Gln Gln Gln Gln Gln Gln

Codon number:

36	37	38	39	40	41	42	43	44	45	46	47	48	49	50

DNA:

CAG CAG CAG CAG CAG CCG CCA CCG CCG CCG CCG CCG CCG CCG CCT

RNA:

CAG CAG CAG CAG CAG CCG CCA CCG CCG CCG CCG CCG CCG CCG CCU

Protein:

Gln Gln Gln Gln Gln Pro Pro Pro Pro Pro Pro Pro Pro Pro Pro

The insert has the following sequence: $(Gln)_{34}$.

The normal protein has a sequence that contains 23 glutamines. Your patient has 34 extra glutamines in this region for a total of 57 glutamines. We do not know the function of the 23 glutamines in the protein, which is known as *huntingtin*. The fact that the long polyglutamine molecule binds to the enzyme glyceraldehyde-3-phosphate dehydrogenase whereas the shorter polyglutamine does not suggests that the mutated protein may impair the glycolytic pathway.

Various drugs that inhibit mitochondrial energy metabolism lead, in animals, to the same symptoms exhibited by your patient, suggesting that impaired energy metabolism may be the problem.

The association of huntingtin with vesicles suggests that it may be involved in synaptic vesicle transport, a process very important for neuronal function and one that requires energy.

b. The brain is uniquely dependent on glucose metabolism. Other tissues can burn fat, but the brain requires glucose. A blockage of the glycolytic pathway, in which the enzyme glyceraldehyde-3-phosphate dehydrogenase is located, would thus be very serious for the brain.

In addition, huntingtin interacts with a protein (presently known as protein X) that is enriched in the brain. This could be irrelevant to the etiology of the disease, but, on the other hand, one could also speculate that protein X may potentiate the deleterious effect of the mutation.

c. Long stretches of glutamine have a tendency to form β-sheets. In addition to the hydrogen bonds between the main-chain amide nitrogen and α-carbonyl oxygens, polyglutamine β-chains contain 50% more hydrogen bonds, these being between their side-chain nitrogens and oxygens. The longer the polyglutamine stretch, the more stable the resulting β-sheet and hence the more likely that it will form. Such β-sheets could interact with other β-sheets in other proteins, such as other molecules of huntingtin to form an aggregate that could precipitate. Alternatively, the mutant huntingtin could bind more tightly to proteins such as glyceraldehyde-3-phosphate dehydrogenase, which is also rich in β-sheets.

d. Ancestry of some of the people with this disease has been traced to individuals living in seventeenth century New England, several of whom were accused of witchcraft. The jerky movements and psychiatric problems associated with this disease could easily be construed by ignorant and superstitious people as demonic possession, a trait supposedly characteristic of witches.

Your patient has HUNTINGTON'S DISEASE.

REFERENCES

Barinaga, M. An intriguing new lead on Huntington's disease. *Science* 271: 1233, 1996.

Beal, M. F. Does impairment of energy metabolism result in excitotoxic neuronal death in neurodegenerative illnesses? *Ann. Neurol.* 31: 119, 1992.

Burke, J. R., Enghild, J. J., Martin, M. E., Jou, Y-S., Myers, R. M., Roses, A. D., Vance, J. M., and Strittmatter, W. J., Huntingtin and DRPLA proteins selectively interact with the enzyme GAPDH. *Nat. Med.* 2: 347, 1996.

DiFiglia, M., Sapp, E., Chase, K., Schwarz, C., Meloni, A., Young, C., Martin, E., Vonsatttel, J.-P., Carraway, R., Reeves, S. A., Boyce, F. M., and Aronin, N. Huntingtin is a cytoplasmic protein associated with vesicles in human and rat brain neurons. *Neuron* 14: 1075, 1995.

Huntington's Disease Collaborative Research Group. A novel gene containing a trinucleotide repeat that is expanded and unstable on Huntongton's disease chromosomes. *Cell* 72: 971, 1993.

Li, X.-J., Li, S.-H., Sharp, A. H., Nucifora, F. C., Schilling, G., Lanahan, A., Worley, P., Snyder, S. H., and Ross, C. A. A Huntington-associated protein enriched in brain with implications for pathology. *Nature* 378: 398, 1995.

Perutz, M. F., Johnson, T., Suzuki, M., and Finch, J. T. Glutamine repeats as polar zippers: their possible role in inherited neurodegenerative diseases. *Proc. Natl. Acad. Sci. USA* 91: 5355, 1994.

Sharp, A. H., Loev, S. J., Schilling, G., Li, S.-H., Li, X.-J., Bao, J., Wagster, M. V., Kotzuk, J. A., Steiner, J. P., Lo, A., Hedreen, J., Sisodia, S., Snyder, S. H., Dawson, T. M., Ryugo, D. K., and Ross, C. A. Widespread expression of Huntington's disease gene (IT15) protein product. *Neuron* 14: 1065, 1995.

Stott, K., Blackburn, J. M., Butler, P. J. G., and Perutz, M. Incorporation of glutamine repeats makes protein oligomerize: implications for neurodegenerative diseases. *Proc. Natl. Acad. Sci. USA* 92: 6509, 1995.

Vessie, P. R. On the transmission of Huntington's chorea for 300 years—the Bures family group. *J. Nervous Mental Dis.* 76: 553, 1932.

Answer 74

Your protein is apparently a membrane protein since it contains seven transmembrane segments. The altered amino acid is in the sixth segment. Replacing a hydrophobic amino acid with a charged amino acid at this position is likely to be deleterious for the function of the protein, whatever that may be, since the transmembrane segments are largely hydrophobic. As for the function of this protein, the only clue we have to go on is the similarity to the nematode protein, which is located in the membrane of the Golgi and is required for proper interactions of the Golgi with other cellular organelles. One could imagine that your patient's protein may affect the interaction between the Golgi and other cellular structures. In such a case, it is reasonable to speculate that there might be improper processing of proteins that go through the Golgi. One such protein is the β-amyloid precursor protein. Perhaps if the protein lingers too long in the Golgi, some of it may be processed to generate the peptide Aβ, which will precipitate upon secretion. The gradual accumulation of the Aβ plaques will cause deterioration of mental function.

Your patient has EARLY-ONSET FAMILIAL ALZHEIMER'S DISEASE.

This gene, located on chromosome 21, may cause the majority of the early-onset cases of Alzheimer's disease.

REFERENCES

Selkoe, D. J. Missense on the membrane. *Nature* 375: 734, 1995.

Sherrington, R., Rogaev, E. I., Liang, Y., Rogaeva, E. A., Levesque, G., Ikeda, M., Chi, H., Lin, C., Li, G., Holman, K., Tsuda, T., Mar, L., Foncin, J.-F., Bruni, A. C., Montesi, M. P., Sorbi, S., Rainero, I., Pinessi, L., Nee, L., Chumakov, I., Pollen, D., Brookes, A., Sanseau, P., Polinsky, R. J., Wasco, W., Da Silva, H. A. R., Haines, J. L., Pericak-Vance, M. A., Tanzi, R. E., Roses, A. D., Fraser, P. E., Rommens, J. M., and St. George-Hyslop, P. H. Cloning of a gene bearing missense mutations in early-onset familial Alzheimer's disease. *Nature* 365: 754, 1995.

Answer 75

a. There are certain genes whose transcription is increased in the presence of cAMP. These genes contain certain elements in their sequence 29 to 60 base pairs upstream from the site where transcription begins. These elements, which are called cAMP-responsive elements, or CRE, generally contain the sequence TGACG or something similar. The protein CREB (CRE-binding protein) binds to these elements and can stimulate transcription. Your patient's protein is called *CBP*, which stands for *CREB-binding protein*. CBP and CREB operate in a feed-forward loop, where they stimulate production of cAMP-dependent proteins, including protein kinase A, which then phosphorylates CREB, which permits it to interact with CBP and allows for further transcription.

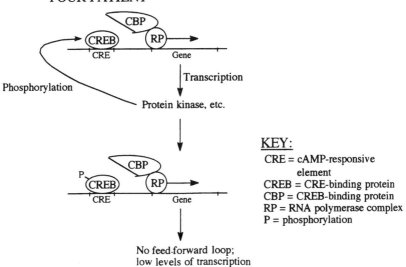

NORMAL PERSON

CBP
CREB RP
CRE   Gene

Phosphorylation

Transcription

Protein kinase, etc.

P CBP
CREB RP
CRE   Gene

More Transcription

YOUR PATIENT

CBP
CREB RP
CRE   Gene

Phosphorylation

Transcription

Protein kinase, etc.

P CBP
CREB RP
CRE   Gene

No feed-forward loop;
low levels of transcription

KEY:
CRE = cAMP-responsive
        element
CREB = CRE-binding protein
CBP = CREB-binding protein
RP = RNA polymerase complex
P = phosphorylation

FIGURE A75-1. **Role of CBP in a normal person and in your patient.** In a normal person (top), CBP connects CREB with the RNA polymerase complex (RP). This allows CREB to stimulate transcription of protein kinases and other proteins. The protein kinase thus produced will phosphorylate CREB, thereby enhancing its activity. This is an example of a feed-forward loop. Your patient lacks a substantial portion of CBP, which can now no longer bind to CREB. Thus, although some transcription of the protein kinase and other genes takes place, there will be no feed-forward loop; even if CREB becomes phosphorylated, its lack of binding to CBP will prevent that phosphorylation from enhancing transcription.

b. The mutation is analyzed as follows:

Codon number:	352	353	354	355	356	357	358	359	360	361	362	363	364	365
Normal person's DNA:	AAA	CTG	ATA	CAG	CAG	CAG	CTG	GTT	CTA	CTG	CTT	CAT	GCT	CAT
Normal person's RNA:	AAA	CUG	AUA	CAG	CAG	CAG	CUG	GUU	CUA	CUG	CUU	CAU	GCU	CAU
Normal person's Lys protein:		Leu	Ilu	Gln	Gln	Gln	Leu	Val	Leu	Leu	Leu	His	Ala	His
Your patient's DNA:	AAA	CTG	ATA	CAG	CAG	TAG	CTG	GTT	CTA	CTG	CTT	CAT	GCT	CAT
Your patient's RNA:	AAA	CUG	AUA	CAG	CAG	UAG	CUG	GUU	CUA	CUG	CUU	CAU	GCU	CAU
Your patient's protein:	Lys	Leu	Ilu	Gln	Gln	STOP								

Your patient's protein has a termination codon at position 357. Since the domain of CBP that binds to CREB is at positions 462 to 661, this entire region will be missing and your patient's CBP will be unable to bind to CREB. This will in turn mean that transcription of the cAMP-responsive elements will be lower than normal. Perhaps some of these elements control differentiation and development in the nervous system. If so, then the symptoms could be explained. It is interesting that in mice, the cAMP pathway plays a role in long-term memory. In the fruit fly *Drosophila*, CREB also plays a role in long-term memory. Although your patient does not have a specific memory problem, these findings in other organisms suggest that cAMP may play a role in mental function.

Your patient has RUBINSTEIN-TAYBI SYNDROME.

REFERENCES

Chrivia, J. C., Kwok, R. P. S., Lamb, N., Hagiwara, M., Montminy, M. R., and Goodman, R. H. Phosphorylated CREB binds specifically to the nuclear protein CBP. *Nature* 365: 855, 1993.

D'Arcangelo, G., and Curran, T. Smart transcription factors. *Nature* 376: 292, 1995.

Goodman, R. H. Regulation of neuropeptide gene expression. *Ann. Rev. Neurosci.* 13: 111, 1990.

Petrij, F., Giles, R. H., Dauwerse, H. G., Saris, J. J., Hennekam, R. C. M., Masuno, M., Tommerup, N., van Ommen, G.-J., Goodman, R. H., Peters, D. J. M., and Breuning, M. H. Rubinstein-Taybi syndrome caused by mutations in the transcriptional co-activator CBP. *Nature* 376: 348, 1995.

Answer 76

a. Alzheimer's disease is caused by abnormal deposition of the Aβ peptide. This deposition can apparently be accelerated greatly by other proteins, but only by certain ones. Albumin has no effect; the apolipoproteins A1 and A2 have no effect. α_1-Antichymotrypsin strongly promotes filament polymerization. Thus, where α_1-antichymotrypsin occurs, you might expect to find amyloid deposits. Also, there is a clear influence of the apolipoprotein E family. Of the three isoforms, E2 by itself has only a small effect. E3 has a larger effect and E4 has a very large one. Interestingly, apolipoprotein E2 appears to inhibit the effect of apolipoprotein E4. It is possible that the Aβ peptide is induced to precipitate by the actions of α_1-antichymotrypsin and apolipoproteins E3 or E4.

There is another intriguing connection between apolipoprotein E and the β-amyloid precursor protein. There is a receptor protein, called *LDL receptor-related protein (LRP)*, which binds to both apolipoprotein E and β-amyloid precursor protein and mediates their endocytosis. The significance of this connection is as yet unclear.

b. The individuals most at risk, based only on the results of this experiment, would be the E4/E4. The ones least at risk would be the E4/E2, since there is even less deposit with E2 and E4 together than with E2 alone. Of course, this experiment does not address the E2/E3 or E3/E4 combinations. Keep in mind that this analysis does not actually consider the cause of excess production of Aβ. This may be the true cause of Alzheimer's. The α_1-antichymotrypsin and the apolipoprotein E4 simply aggravate the problem.

c. The function of the β-amyloid precursor protein is still not known. Perhaps the best clue is that mice that are engineered to lack the protein exhibit decreased activity and decreased muscular strength in their forelimbs. They also had more prominent astrocytes. These findings suggest that the protein may play a role in the organization and function of the nervous system, although it is not yet possible to be more precise. The protein may also play a role in recovery from neuronal injury and in protecting neurons.

REFERENCES

Kounnas, M. Z., Moir, R. D., Rebeck, G. W., Bush, A. I., Argraves, W. S., Tanzi, R. E., Hyman, B. T., and Strickland, D. K. LDL receptor-related protein, a multifunctional ApoE receptor, binds secreted β-amyloid precursor protein and mediates its degradation. *Cell* 82: 331, 1995.

Ma, J., Yee, A., Brewer, H. B., Das, S., and Potter, H. Amyloid-associated proteins α_1-antichymotrypsin and apolipoprotein E promote assembly of Alzheimer β-protein into filaments. *Nature* 372: 92, 1994.

Zheng, H., Jiang, M., Trumbauer, M. E., Sirinathsinghji, D. J. S., Hopkins, R., Smith, D. W., Heavens, R. P., Dawson, G. R., Boyce, S., Conner, M. W., Stevens, K. A., Slunt, H. H., Sisodia, S. S., Chen, H. Y., and Van der Ploeg, L. H. T. β-Amyloid precursor protein-deficient mice show reactive gliosis and decreased locomotor activity. *Cell* 81: 525, 1995.

Answer 77

a. The protein p21^{ras} is a proto-oncogene product. Its role is to stimulate cell proliferation. It is also a type of G protein in that it binds to and slowly hydrolyzes GTP. When it is bound to GTP, p21^{ras} is active. When it is bound to GDP, p21^{ras} is inactive. The protein that is altered in your patient is called *neurofibromin*. The role of neurofibromin is to accelerate the GTPase activity of p21^{ras}. If the neurofibromin is defective, p21^{ras} activity will be too high and excess proliferation results.

b. p21^{ras} is anchored to the membrane by a farnesyl prosthetic group that is transferred to the protein by farnesyltransferase (Fig. A77-1). An inhibitor of the enzyme might inactivate the p21^{ras}, since in the disease this is overactive to begin with.

Your patient has NEUROFIBROMATOSIS TYPE I.

REFERENCES

Basu, T. N., Gutmann, D. H., Fletcher, J. A., Glover, T. W., collins, F. S., and Downward, J. Aberrant regulation of *ras* proteins in malignant tumour cells from type 1 neurofibromatosis patients. *Nature* 356: 713, 1992.

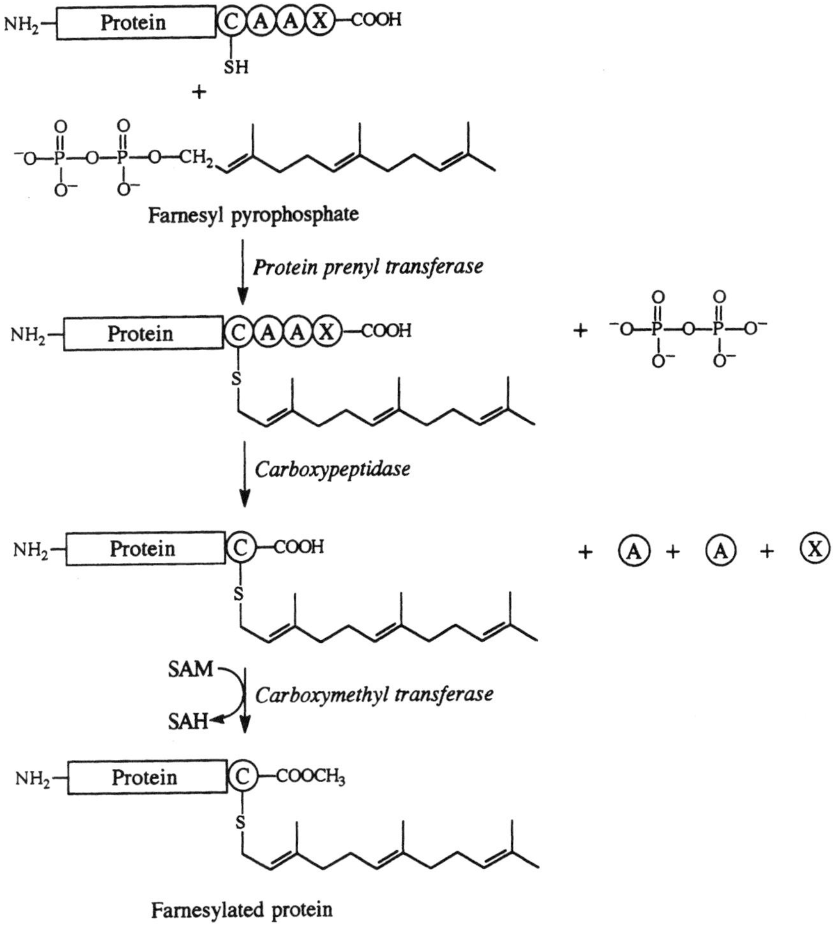

FIGURE A77-1. **Mechanism of protein farnesylation.** In the diagram, C is cysteine, A is any aliphatic amino acid, and X is any amino acid.

Omer, C. A., and Gibbs, J. B. Protein prenylation in eukaryotic microorganisms: Genetics, biology and biochemistry. *Molec. Microbiol.* 11: 219, 1994.

Sinensky, M., and Lutz, R. J. The prenylation of proteins. *BioEssays* 14: 25, 1992.

Yan, N., Ricca, C., Fletcher, J., Glover, T., Seizinger, B. R., and Manne, V. Farnesyltransferase inhibitors block the neurofibromatosis type I (NF1) malignant phenotype. *Cancer Res.* 55: 3569, 1995.

Answer 78

The mutation is analyzed as follows:

Codon number:	54	55	56	57	58	59	60
Normal person's DNA:	CTG	GGC	CTC	CGA	GAA	ACC	TGG
Normal person's RNA:	CUG	GGC	CUC	CGA	GAA	ACC	UGG
Normal person's protein:	Leu	Gly	Leu	Arg	Glu	Thr	Trp
Your patient's DNA:	CTG	GGC	CTC	TGA	GAA	ACC	TGG
Your patient's RNA:	CUG	GGC	CUC	UGA	GAA	ACC	UGG
Your patient's protein:	Leu	Gly	Leu	STOP			

There is a termination codon at position 57 in your patient's protein from his tumor cells. Whatever that protein is doing, it is probably completely nonfunctional as a result of being deprived of the last 90% of its sequence because of this mutation.

Ezrin and moesin are proteins that connect integral membrane proteins, such as integrins, to the cytoskeleton. They thus help mediate processes such as cell migration and contact inhibition. If your patient's protein is similar to these, then its job may be the same. Loss of that protein in the cells in which it is normally expressed may cause those cells to migrate abnormally and, perhaps most important, lose their ability to undergo contact inhibition. Without contact inhibition, the cells could keep proliferating. The altered protein is called *merlin* or *schwannomin*.

Your patient has NEUROFIBROMATOSIS TYPE 2.

REFERENCES

Kreis, T., and Vale, R. (Eds.). *Guidebook to the Cytoskeletal and Motor Proteins*, Oxford: Oxford University Press, 1993.

Rouleau, G. R., Merel, P., Lutchman, M., Sanson, M., Zucman, J., Marineau, C., Hoang-Xuan, K., Demczuk, S., Desmaze, C., Plougastel, B., Pulst, S. M., Lenoir, G., Bijlsma, E., Fashold, R., Dumanski, J., de Jong, P., Parry, D., Eldrige, R., Aurias, A., Delattre, O., and Thomas, G. Alteration in a new gene encoding a putative membrane-organizing protein causes neurofibromatosis type 2. *Nature* 363: 515, 1993.

Trofatter, J. A., MacCollin, M. M., Rutter, J. L., Murrell, J. R., Duyao, M. P., Parry, D. M., Eldridge, R., Kley, N., Menon, A. G., Pulaski, K., Haase, V. H., Ambrose, C. M., Munroe, D., Bove, C., Haines, J. L., Martuza, R. L., MacDonald, M. E.,

Seizinger, B. R., Short, M. P., Buckler, A. J., and Gusella, J. F. A novel moesin-, ezrin, radixin-like gene is a candidate for the neurofibromatosis 2 tumor suppressor. *Cell* 72: 791, 1993.

Answer 79

The mutation is analyzed as follows:

Codon number:	139	140	141	142	143
Normal person's DNA:	GTG	GTG	TTC	CGG	CTG
Normal person's RNA:	GUG	GUG	UUC	CGG	CUG
Normal person's protein:	Val	Val	Phe	Arg	Leu
Your patient's DNA:	GTG	GTG	TTC	TGG	CTG
Your patient's RNA:	GUG	GUG	UUC	UGG	CUG
Your patient's protein:	Val	Val	Phe	Trp	Leu

Your patient has a tryptophan at position 142 instead of an arginine. This is in one of the transmembrane domains of the protein. Connexin 32 is one of the gap junction proteins. Gap junctions, found in various cell types, are tiny pores in the cell membranes of two adjacent cells that permit direct communication between the two cells. Replacing the arginine by a tryptophan is likely to alter the conformation of the transmembrane helix in such a way as to close the pore. Thus, the communication between the two cells will cease. Gap junctions, although found in quite a few tissues, seem to be critical for proper function of Schwann cells. Apparently, if they are not working properly, this could result in degeneration of the Schwann cells and improper myelination of the neurons, leading to loss of neural function.

Your patient has CHARCOT-MARIE-TOOTH DISEASE.

REFERENCES

Ballabio, A., and Zoghbi, H. Y. Charcot-Marie-Tooth disease and hereditary neuropathy with liability to pressure palsies. C. R. Scriver, A. L. Beaudet, W. S. Sly, D. Valle, J. B. Stanbury, J. B. Wyngaarden, and D. S. Fredrickson (Eds.). *The Metabolic and Molecular Bases of Inherited Disease*. New York: McGraw-Hill, 1995, Vol. III, Chap. 154C, p. 4569.

Bennett, M. V. L. Connexins in disease. *Nature* 368: 18, 1994.

Bergoffen, J., Scherer, S. S., Wang, S., Oronzi Scott, M., Bone, L. J., Chen, P. K., Lensch, M. W., Chance, P. F., and Fischbeck, K. H. Connexin mutations in X-linked Charcot-Marie-Tooth disease. *Science* 262: 2039, 1993.

Answer 80

a. If the immunoglobulin G fraction was able to evoke an electric potential in a cultured neuron, then something in that fraction must be acting like an agonist to a neurotransmitter. To what kind of neurotransmitter? The fact that it is blocked by 6-cyano-7-nitro-quinoxaline-2,3-dione, a known agonist of glutamate, suggests that the neurotransmitter is glutamate. This is corroborated by the finding that the same symptoms can be induced in rabbits by injection with the glutamate R3 receptor. The immunoglobulin G fraction contains antibodies. Your patient must have an antibody against her glutamate R3 receptors. She is suffering from an autoimmune disease. The antibody, however, is not acting to inactivate, but to activate, the receptor. Thus, it is as if a constant high level of glutamate is being produced in the central nervous system.

b. Plasma exchange, to get rid of the antibodies, at least temporarily, would be a good treatment. As a matter of fact, it has produced dramatic improvement in this condition.

Your patient has RASMUSSEN'S ENCEPHALITIS.

REFERENCES

Barinaga, M. Antibodies linked to rare epilepsy. *Science* 268: 362, 1995.

Rogers, S. W., Andrews, P. I., Gahring, L. C., Whisenand, T., Cauley, K., Crain, B., Hughes, T. E., Heinemann, S. F., and McNamara, J. O. Autoantibodies to glutamate receptor GluR3 in Rasmussen's encephalitis. *Science* 265: 648, 1994.

Twyman, R. E., Gahring, L. C., Spiess, J., and Rogers, S. W. Glutamate receptor antibodies activate a subset of receptors and reveal an agonist binding site. *Neuron* 14: 755, 1995.

Problem 81

Your patient is a 45-year-old male convict with a long criminal history, including exhibitionism, rape, and arson. In his urine he has elevated levels of normetanephrine and tyramine and decreased levels of 5-hydroxyindole-3-acetic acid, homovanillic acid, and vanillylmandelic acid. You find that he has an altered gene. Codon 296 in this gene is TAG instead of CAG.

You have heard that rats deprived of REM sleep are much more inclined to fight if they are also given apomorphine. Another experiment, done with humans, indicated that administration of clorgyline almost completely suppressed their REM sleep.

a. What protein is defective in your patient?

b. How might the mutation play a role in his criminal history?

Problem 82

Your patient has dilated blood vessels in the whites of his eyes. He has a tendency to make jerking movements. He also has glucose intolerance. In addition, he often gets lung infections and is hypersensitive to X-rays. His mother and sister have had breast cancer. You have found that he has a deletion in a gene. You do not know the function of the protein encoded by the gene, but you observe that it is similar in sequence to the catalytic subunit of another protein, phosphatidylinositol-3'-kinase. It also resembles a yeast protein called Mec1.

Based on this information, speculate on how the defective protein can cause the symptoms you have observed.

Problem 83

Your patient is an epileptic with some muscle weakness and progressive dementia. He is also losing his hearing. His mother and his maternal grandmother also had the disease. You do a biopsy and purify his mitochondrial DNA. You find that he has a mutation at nucleotide position 8344, in which an A is replaced by a G. When you analyze his mitochondrial tRNA content, you find that the level of tRNA^{Lys} is 65% of the normal. The polycistronic RNA containing this tRNA^{Lys} as well as other tRNAs is present at normal levels. Purifying the tRNA^{Lys} and incubating it with aminoacyl-tRNA synthetases and radioactive lysine, you find that attachment of lysine is about 45% of normal. Attachment of CCA to the tRNA^{Lys} is normal. Protein synthesis was severely depressed in these mitochondria. Among the products of protein synthesis were fragments of subunits of cytochrome oxidase and cytochrome b.

Based on this information, show how the mutation causes the symptoms and the experimental findings.

Problem 84

One of your patients (patient A) is a 2-year-old boy who suffers from very poor coordination. He has constant involuntary movement of his eyeballs.

You find that he has an alteration in the gene for lipophilin. The alteration is shown here:

Codon number:	135	136	137	138	139	140	141	142	143
Normal person:	GAG	CGG	GTG	TGT	CAT	TGT	TTG	GGA	AAA
Your patient:	GAG	CGG	GTG	TGT	TAT	TGT	TTG	GGA	AAA

a. Describe the expression of the lipophilin gene.

b. How might the mutation lead to the observed defect?

c. A second patient (patient B) has an alteration in which tryptophan at position 162 is replaced by an arginine. He has the same symptoms as your first patient. In addition, he has overall poor muscle tone and is mentally retarded. Why are his symptoms so much more severe than your other patient's?

Problem 85

Your patient is a 12-year-old girl with gradually increasing symptoms. These began with a twisting of the foot and and then spread to the hands. The symptoms are at their worst at night and at their best in the early morning after she wakes up. You draw some blood and you prepare some lymphocytes. From these you make a cell-free extract and add GTP and measure the production of 7,8-dihydroneopterin triphosphate, which you find to be 7% of normal.

a. What is the defective enzyme in your patient?

b. How does this defect lead to the disease?

c. How would you treat this patient?

Problem 86

Your patient is mentally retarded; he is unable to speak in comprehensible words. He has a shuffling gait and adducted thumbs. He has a gene with an altered sequence, shown here:

Codon number:	596	597	598	599
Normal person:	GAA	CTG	GAT	GTG
Your patient:	GAA	CTG	AAT	GTG

The protein encoded by this gene has an extracellular portion, a transmembrane portion and a cytoplasmic portion. The extracellular domain is subdivided into six immunoglobulin type C2 domains and five fibronectin type III domains. Position 598 is highly conserved in evolution and is located in one of the immunoglobulin-type domains in the loop between two strands of a β-sheet and seven residues after a cysteine involved in a disulfide bridge.

a. What is the likely role of this protein?

b. How might the mutation cause the observed symptoms?

Problem 87

Your patient is an 8-year-old boy who became blind shortly after birth, then underwent rapid mental deterioration until, at the age of 3, his electroencephalogram became flat. You obtain cells from him and do an assay in which you add Hras protein labeled with radioactive palmitate; you measure the release of radioactive palmitate. You find that activity is 2% that which you would expect to find in cells from a normal individual.

Your patient has an altered gene. The alteration is shown here:

Codon number: 119   120   121   122   123   124   125
Normal person: CAA TTT CTG AGG GCA GTG GCT
Your patient: CAA TTT CTG TGG GCA GTG GCT

a. What is the defective enzyme?

b. How might the mutation lead to the enzyme defect?

Problem 88

Your patient has several brief seizures almost every night. The seizures typically begin shortly after he falls asleep, although sometimes they occur later in the night. Occasionally, he takes a nap during the day and has a seizure at that time. His seizures began when he was 5 years old and have been occurring ever since. During his seizures he exhibits jerky movements and his eyes roll up. The attacks often begin with a feeling of a cramp in one leg. Electroencephalograms you do of your patient during his seizures suggest that the greatest activity is in the frontal lobe.

You purify, clone, and sequence the gene for his neuronal nicotinic acetylcholine receptor α4 subunit and find that it contains a mutation. Here is the partial sequence, compared to that of a normal individual:

Codon number:	242	243	244	245	246	247	248	249	250
Normal person:	AAG	ATC	ACG	CTG	TGC	ATC	TCC	GTG	CTG
Your patient:	AAG	ATC	ACG	CTG	TGC	ATC	TTC	GTG	CTG

A search of the literature reveals some sequences in other acetylcholine receptors:

Rat α1:	Lys	Met	Thr	Leu	Ser	Ilu	Ser	Val	Leu
Rat α7:	Lys	Ilu	Ser	Leu	Gly	Ilu	Thr	Val	Leu
Chicken α2:	Lys	Ilu	Thr	Leu	Cys	Ilu	Ser	Val	Leu
Xenopus:	Lys	Ilu	Thr	Leu	Ser	Val	Ser	Val	Leu
Electric eel:	Lys	Met	Thr	Leu	Ser	Ilu	Ser	Val	Leu
Drosophila:	Lys	Ilu	Ala	Leu	Cys	Ilu	Ser	Ilu	Leu

a. How does the mutation lead to the disease?

b. Speculate on why the seizures are associated with sleep and localized to the frontal lobe?

Problem 89

Your patient is a 5-year-old girl who is deaf in both ears and suffers from severe constipation. She also has patches of skin and hair with no pigmentation. You find a change in her gene for preproendothelin-3. The change is as follows:

Codon number:	156	157	158	159	160
Normal person:	CAC	TTG	CGC	TGC	GCT
Your patient:	CAC	TTG	CGC	TTC	GCT

a. Speculate on how the mutation leads to the disease.

A possible clue is that preproendothelin-3 has cysteines at the following positions (among others): 97, 99, 107, 111, 159, 161, 169, and 173.

b. How is preproendothelin-3 processed?

c. If endothelin-3 and endothelin-1 have the same receptors, why do they have very different actions?

Answer 81

a. The metabolites in the urine suggest that your patient has a deficiency with monoamine oxidase. There are two kinds of monoamine oxidase: monoamine oxidase A, which preferentially converts normetanephrine to vanillylmandelate, and serotonin to

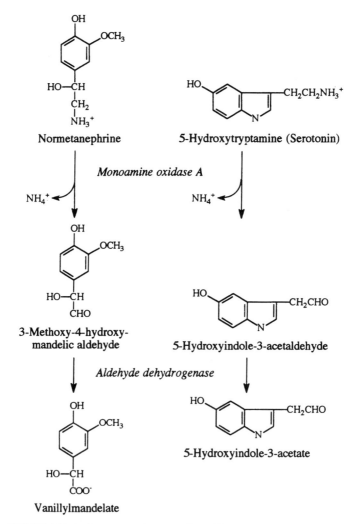

FIGURE A81-1. **Some reactions catalyzed by monoamine oxidase A.**

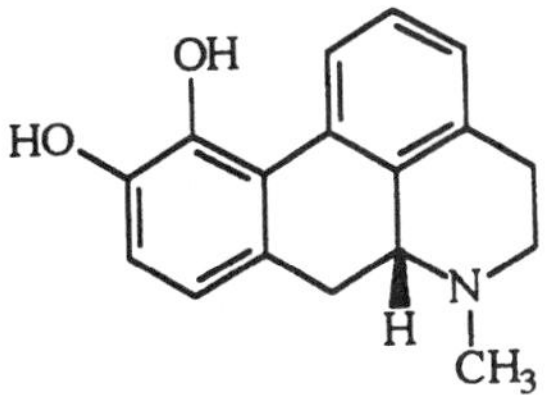

FIGURE A81-2. **Structures of apomorphine and clorgyline.**

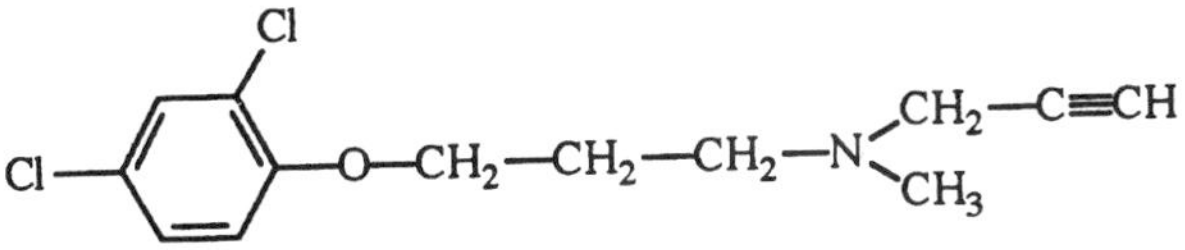

5-hydroxyindole-3-acetaldehyde, which is metabolized to 5-hydroxyindole-3-acetic acid (Fig. A81-1), and monoamine oxidase B, which prefers phenylethylamine and benzylamine. In fact, the defective enzyme is *monoamine oxidase A*.

b. Your patient has a termination codon at position 296 instead of a glutamine codon. Thus, he is likely to have a defective monoamine oxidase A. Inhibitors of this enzyme, such as clorgyline (Fig. A81-2), have been shown to suppress REM sleep. Conceivably, since he lacks the enzyme, he will also have less than normal REM sleep. Since he lacks the enzyme, he will have elevated levels of dopamine. Apomorphine (Fig. A81-2) is a dopamine agonist, which stimulates dopaminergic receptors. Thus, his situation may replicate the experiment with rats in which deprivation of REM sleep combined with dopaminergic stimulation induced aggressive behavior.

REFERENCES

Brunner, H. G., Nelen, M., Breakefield, X. O., Ropers, H. H., and van Oost, B. A. Abnormal behavior associated with a point mutation in the structural gene for monoamine oxidase A. *Science* 262, 578, 1993.

Cohen, R. M., Pickar, D., Garnett, D., Lipper, S., Gillin, J. C., and Murphy, D. L.

REM sleep suppression induced by selective monoamine oxidase inhibitors. *Psychopharmacology* 78: 137, 1982.

Johnston, J. P. Some observations upon a new inhibitor of monoamine oxidase in brain tissue. *Biochem. Pharmacol.* 17: 1285, 1968.

Tufik, S., Lindsey, C. J., and Carlini, E. A. Does REM sleep deprivation induce a supersensitivity of dopaminergic receptors in the rat brain? *Pharmacology* 16: 98, 1978.

Answer 82

Your patient's protein resembles the catalytic subunit of phosphatidylinositol-3'-kinase (PIK) (Fig. A82-1). If your patient's protein has a similar function, then it plays a key role in signal transduction. For example, the tyrosine kinase activated in the insulin receptor phosphorylates proteins that interact with PIK. A defect in PIK may make cells resistant to insulin, leading to glucose intolerance. Neuronal cells appear to require certain growth factors for their continued health. PIK plays a role in this pathway as well. A loss of PIK activity could lead to death of some neurons in the cerebellum and hence to the jerking movements and lack of coordination. The same PIK pathway is involved in activation of T cells by interleukin-2; thus, loss of PIK activity could lead to numerous infections.

The yeast protein Mec1 is responsible for protecting yeast cells against radiation damage. It is possible that your patient's protein is a cell cycle control protein that acts like Mec1 to shut down the cell cycle in cells with damaged DNA, thereby giving repair enzymes a chance to fix the damage. A defect in a protein like that may allow the cells to continue replicating with the damaged DNA, thereby giving rise to mutant cells, many of which will die and cause lesions. People with a single copy of this defective gene, such as your patient's mother and sister, lack many of the symptoms but have a higher susceptibility to breast cancer. Perhaps the same principle operates here, namely, that a defective protein may allow damaged DNA to replicate and that may lead to tumor formation.

The origin of the dilated blood vessels in his eyes is unclear. Conceivably, this could be due to abnormal response to a growth factor.

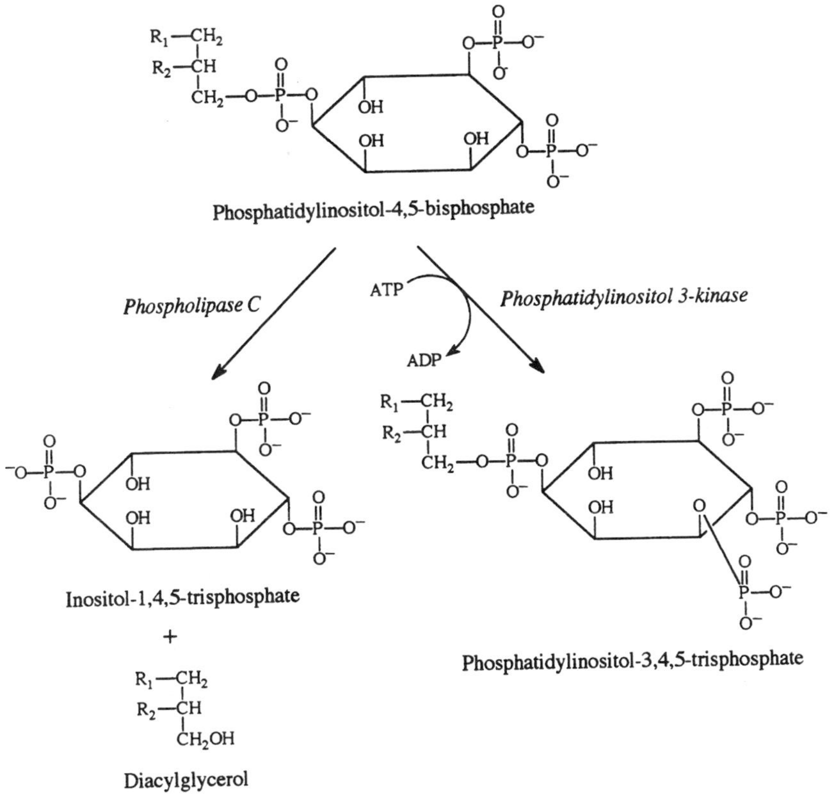

FIGURE A82-1. **Phosphatidyl 3-kinase reaction.** The figure also shows how this reaction is connected to the synthesis of inositol-1,4,5-trisphosphate.

Your patient has ATAXIA TELANGIECTASIA.

REFERENCES

Burgering, B. M. T., and Coffer, P. J. Protein kinase B (c-Akt) in phosphatidylinositol-3OH kinase signal transduction. *Nature* 376: 599, 1995.

Downward, J. A target for PI(3) kinase. *Nature* 376: 553, 1995.

Nowak, R. Discovery of AT gene sparks biomedical research bonanza. *Science* 268: 1700, 1995.

Savitsky, K., Bar-Shira, A., Gilad, S., Rotman, G., Ziv, Y., Vanagaite, L., Tagle, D. A., Smith, S., Uziel, T., Sfez, S., Ashkenazi, M., Pecker, I., Frydman, M., Harnik, R., Patanjali, S. R., Simmons, A., Clines, G. A., Sartiel, A., Gatti, R. A.,

Chessa, L., Sanal, O., Lavin, M. F., Jaspers, N. G. J., Taylor, M. R., Arlett, C. F., Miki, T., Weissman, S. M., Lovett, M., Collins, F. S., and Shiloh, Y. A single ataxia telangiectasia gene with a product similar to PI-3 kinase. *Science* 268: 1749, 1995.

Answer 83

The mutation at position 8344 is in the gene coding for tRNA^{Lys}. (This gene consists of nucleotides 8295 to 8364). The mutation is in the highly conserved TΨC loop of the tRNA^{Lys}. It is not in the anticodon loop nor in the aminoacyl stem. Nor is CCA attachment affected. Furthermore, the mutation does not affect the polycistronic RNA; hence, it must be acting at the level of the tRNA^{Lys} itself. Thus, the tRNA^{Lys} is physically able to react with lysine and it should recognize the codon for lysine, but it does not get charged normally. The most probable interpretation is that this mutation destabilizes the tRNA^{Lys} and diminishes its affinity for the aminoacyl-tRNA synthetase. Also, the destabilization causes it to be degraded by nucleases. Thus, the level of tRNA^{Lys} bound to lysine in these mitochondria is very low. The result will be serious flaws in protein synthesis, in which incomplete proteins will be made. The consequence of this will be mitochondria whose electron transport and oxidative phosphorylation function is impaired.

Your patient has MYOCLONUS EPILEPSY WITH RAGGED RED FIBERS.

REFERENCES

Enriquez, J. A., Chomyn, A., and Attardi, G. MtDNA mutation in MERRF syndrome causes defective aminoacylation of tRNA^{Lys} and premature translation termination. *Nat. Genet.* 10: 47, 1995.

Shoffner, J. M., and Wallace, D. C. Oxidative phosphorylation diseases. C. R. Scriver, A. L. Beaudet, W. S. Sly, D. Valle, J. B. Stanbury, J. B. Wyngaarden, and D. S. Fredrickson (Eds.). *The Metabolic and Molecular Bases of Inherited Disease.* New York: McGraw-Hill, 1995, Vol. I, Chap. 46, p. 1535–1609.

Answer 84

a. The lipophilin gene is expressed as two alternatively spliced proteins (Fig. A84-1). One is called lipophilin (or proteolipid protein); the other is called DM20. Lipophilin is 276 residues in length; DM20 is identical to lipophilin, except that residues 116 to 150 have been deleted. Serine 198 has an attached fatty acid (16:0, 18:0, or 18:1). Lipophilin is expressed later and is involved in myelin sheet compaction, while DM20 is expressed by oligodendrocytes and in developing brain. Patient A's mutation, in exon 3B, produces mutant lipophilin but normal DM20.

b. The mutation is analyzed as follows:

Codon number:	135	136	137	138	139	140	141	142	143
Normal person's DNA:	GAG	CGG	GTG	TGT	CAT	TGT	TTG	GGA	AAA
Normal person's RNA:	GAG	CGG	GUG	UGU	CAU	UGU	UUG	GGA	AAA
Normal person's protein:	Glu	Arg	Val	Cys	His	Cys	Leu	Gly	Lys
Your patient's DNA:	GAG	CGG	GTG	TGT	TAT	TGT	TTG	GGA	AAA
Your patient's RNA:	GAG	CGG	GUG	UGU	UAU	UGU	UUG	GGA	AAA
Your patient's protein:	Glu	Arg	Val	Cys	Tyr	Cys	Leu	Gly	Lys

Patient A's lipophilin has a tyrosine at position 139 instead of a histidine. This is in the intracellular domain. The precise function of this domain is not clear. However, this mutation replaces a polar residue with a hydrophobic residue; such a mutation is likely to alter the conformation of this region and be deleterious for its function.

c. There are two reasons why patient B has more severe symptoms: (1) The second patient's mutation is in a transmembrane helix. Replacing a hydrophobic tryptophan with a highly polar arginine is bound to alter the conformation of the helix if not destroy it altogether, since a charged residue may not be stable in a transmembrane domain. (2) Patient A has a mutation at position 139, which is in the segment that is deleted in the DM20 product, although not in lipophilin. Patient B has a mutation at position 162, which is present in both DM20 and lipophilin. Thus, patient A has normal DM20 while patient B does not; both patients have mutat-

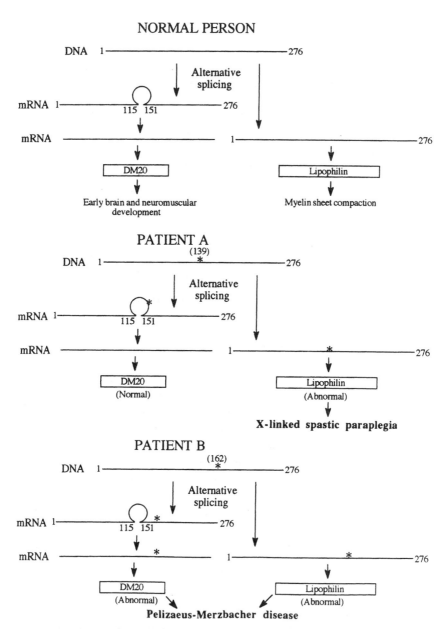

FIGURE A84-1. **Synthesis of lipophilin and DM20.** In a normal person (top), DM20 and lipophilin are made by alternative splicing from a single gene. In patient A (middle), the mutation at codon 139 is excised in DM20 although not in lipophilin, so patient A has a milder disease. In patient B (middle), the mutation at codon 161 is expressed in both gene products, leading to more severe disease.

ed lipophilin. Since DM20 plays a bigger role in development than does lipophilin, your second patient is likely to have more severe problems because much of the development of the nervous system will be affected.

Patient A has X-LINKED SPASTIC PARAPLEGIA; Patient B has PELIZAEUS-MERZBACHER DISEASE.

REFERENCES

Diehl, H.-J., Schaich, M., Budzinski, R.-M., and Stoffel, W. Individual exons encode the integral membrane domains of human myelin proteolipid protein. *Proc. Natl. Acad. Sci. USA* 83: 9807, 1986.

Hudson, L. D., Puckett, C., Berndt, J., Chan, J., and Gencic, S. Mutation of the proteolipid protein gene *PLP* in a human X chromosome-linked myelin disorder. *Proc. Natl. Acad. Sci. USA* 86: 8128, 1989.

Nave, K.-A., Lai, C., Bloom, F. E., and Milner, R. J. Splice site selection in the proteolipid protein (PLP) gene transcript and primary structure of the DM-20 protein of central nervous system myelin. *Proc. Natl. Acad. Sci. USA* 84: 5665, 1987.

Popot, J.-L., Pham Dinh, D., and Dautigny, A. Major myelin proteolipid: The 4-α-helix topology. *J. Membrane Biol.* 120: 233, 1991.

Saugier-Veber, P., Munnich, A., Bonneau, D., Rozet, J.-M., Le Merrer, M., Gil, R., and Boespflug-Tanguy, O. X-linked spastic paraplegia and Pelizaeus-Merzbacher disease are allelic disorders at the proteolipid protein locus. *Nat. Genet.* 6: 257, 1994.

Zoghbi, H. Y., and Ballabio, A. Pelizaeus-Merzbacher disease. In C. R. Scriver, A. L. Beaudet, W. S. Sly, D. Valle, J. B. Stanbury, J. B. Wyngaarden, and D. S. Fredrickson (Eds.). *The Metabolic and Molecular Bases of Inherited Disease.* New York: McGraw-Hill, 1995, Vol. III, Chap. 154E, p. 4581.

Answer 85

a. The defective enzyme converts GTP to 7,8-dihydro-neopterin triphosphate (Fig. A85-1). This enzyme is *GTP cyclohydrolase I*. This enzyme catalyzes the rate-limiting step in the biosynthesis of tetrahydrobiopterin.

b. With the enzyme having less activity, less tetrahydrobiopterin is made. Tetrahydrobiopterin is a cofactor for three enzymes (Fig. A85-2): phenylalanine hydroxylase, tyrosine hydroxy-

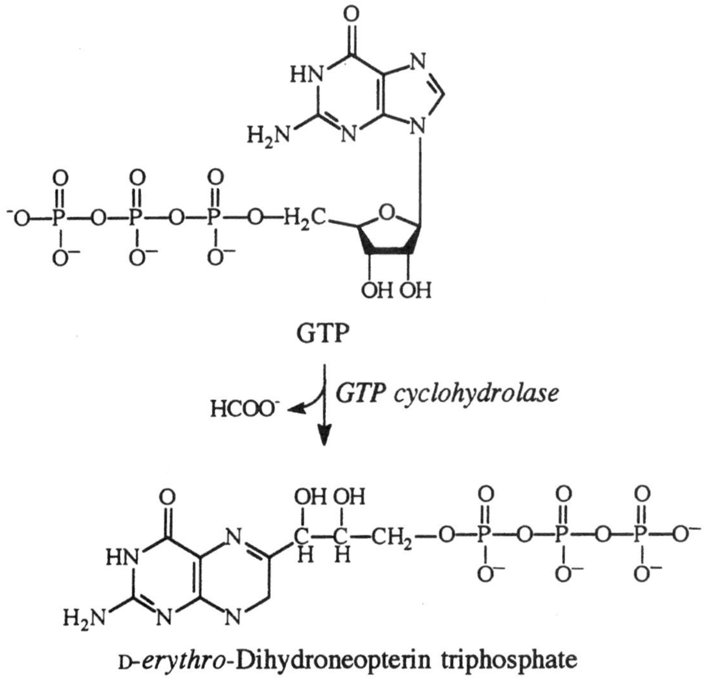

GTP

HCOO⁻ ◄— GTP cyclohydrolase

D-*erythro*-Dihydroneopterin triphosphate

FIGURE A85-1. **GTP cyclohydrolase reaction.** The full pathway for tetrahydro-biopterin biosynthesis is given in Learning Biochemistry, Figure A1-2.

lase, and tryptophan hydroxylase. These three enzymes catalyze, respectively, the conversion of phenylalanine to tyrosine, of tyrosine to 3,4-dihydroxyphenylalanine (L-DOPA), which is a precursor of dopamine, and of tryptophan to 5-hydroxytryptophan, which is a precursor of serotonin. Lack of cofactor might affect all of these reactions, but your patient's symptoms suggest that he lacks dopamine. At night when he is asleep, your patient is not drawing so much on his dopamine reserves, which can be built up by the pathway, which functions slowly with the defective GTP cyclohydrolase I. That is why his symptoms are at their best in the morning and at their worst at night.

c. The indicated treatment is L-DOPA, which could substitute for the L-DOPA he is only able to make in small quantities. This is

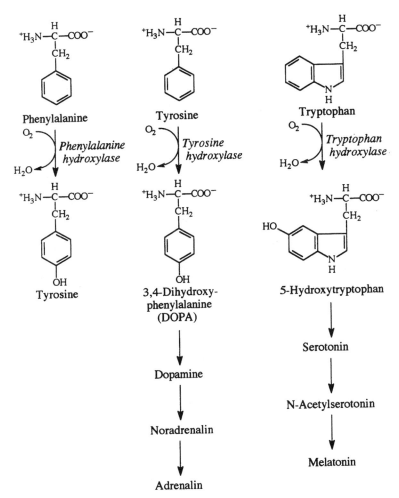

FIGURE A85-2. **Three reactions catalyzed by enzymes requiring tetrahydro-biopterin co-factor.** As you can see in the figure, tyrosine hydroxylase leads to the synthesis of the catecholamines, while tryptophan hydroxylase leads to synthesis of serotonin and melatonin.

also the treatment for Parkinson's disease, which also is caused by lack of dopamine biosynthesis.

Your patient has HEREDITARY PROGRESSIVE DYSTONIA WITH MARKED DIURNAL FLUCTUATION.

REFERENCES

Ichinose, H., Ohye, T., Takahashi, E., Seki, N., Hori, T., Segawa, M., Nomura, Y., Endo, K., Tanaka, H., Tsuji, S., Fujita, K., and Nagatsu, T. Hereditary progressive dystonia with marked diurnal fluctuation caused by mutations in the GTP cyclohydrolase I gene. *Nat. Genet.* 8: 236, 1994.

Answer 86

a. This protein, containing the immunoglobulin-like and fibronectin-like domains sounds like an adhesion protein. In fact it is called *L1CAM* (*L1 cell adhesion protein*). Presumably, L1CAM is involved in recognition of components of the matrix or perhaps proteins attached to other cells. Probably its role is to arrange that neurons grow properly.

b. The mutation is analyzed as follows:

Codon number:	596	597	598	599
Normal person's DNA:	GAA	CTG	GAT	GTG
Normal person's RNA:	GAA	CUG	GAU	GUG
Normal person's protein:	Glu	Leu	Asp	Val
Your patient's DNA:	GAA	CTG	AAT	GTG
Your patient's RNA:	GAA	CUG	AAU	GUG
Your patient's protein:	Glu	Leu	Asn	Val

Your patient's L1CAM has an asparagine acid at position 598 instead of an aspartic acid. This replaces a negatively charged amino acid with a neutral one. This is potentially a serious change since this aspartic acid is highly conserved. One could imagine that introducing a neutral residue into this position could rearrange the β-sheet and move the nearby cysteine. If this should happen, perhaps the right combination of disulfide bridges would not form and the protein might become unstable or simply not interact correctly with its as yet unknown target. In either case, the mutation would interfere with proper cell adhesion in the developing nervous system, and this would cause the mental retardation and other symptoms.

Your patient has **MASA SYNDROME** (MASA = *m*ental retardation, *a*phasia, *s*huffling gait, and *a*dducted thumbs).

REFERENCES

Jouet, M., Rosenthal, A., Armstrong, G., MacFarlane, J., Stevenson, R., Paterson, J., Metzenberg, A., Ionasescu, V., Temple, K., and Kenwrick, S. X-linked spastic paraplegia (SPG1), MASA syndrome and X-linked hydrocephalus result from mutations in the *L1* gene. *Nat. Genet.* 7: 402, 1994.

Vits, L., Van Camp, G., Coucke, P., Fransen, E., de Boulle, K., Reyniers, E., Korn, B., Poustka, A., Wilson, G., Schrander-Stumpel, C., Winter, R. M., Schwartz, C., and Willems, P. J. MASA syndrome is due to mutations in the neural cell adhesion gene *L1CAM*. *Nat. Genet.* 7: 408, 1994.

Answer 87

a. The defective enzyme is *palmitoyl protein thioesterase*. This enzyme catabolizes palmitoyl protein complexes (Fig. A87-1).

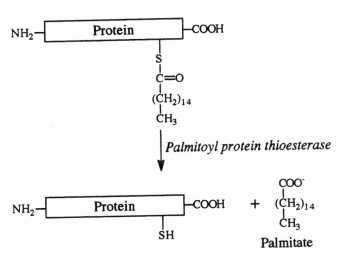

FIGURE A87-1. **Palmitoyl protein thioesterase reaction.**

b. The mutation is analyzed as follows:

Codon number:	119	120	121	122	123	124	125
Normal person's DNA:	CAA	TTT	CTG	AGG	GCA	GTG	GCT
Normal person's RNA:	CAA	UUU	CUG	AGG	GCA	GUG	GCU
Normal person's protein:	Gln	Phe	Leu	Arg	Ala	Val	Ala
Your patient's DNA:	CAA	TTT	CTG	TGG	GCA	GTG	GCT
Your patient's RNA:	CAA	UUU	CUG	UGG	GCA	GUG	GCU
Your patient's protein:	Gln	Phe	Leu	Trp	Ala	Val	Ala

Your patient has a tryptophan at position 122 instead of an arginine. Although it is not certain what the structure of the enzyme is, replacing a strongly polar amino acid such as arginine with a very hydrophobic amino acid such as tryptophan is very likely to cause alterations in the structure. For example, if the arginine was on the interior of the molecule, it probably engaged in an electrostatic bond. The tryptophan that replaced it cannot do so. Thus, whatever stability this bond contributed to the structure is lost. If the arginine was not in an electrostatic bond, then it was probably on the exterior of the protein. The tryptophan that replaces it would most likely move more into the interior of the protein, thereby changing the conformation.

How an inactive palmitoyl protein thioesterase results in the disease is not clear. Conceivably, a protein involved in regulation of neuronal growth or function may need to be released from its membrane anchor in order to do its job. Since catalysis of this release could be the role of the palmitoyl protein thioesterase, lack of this enzyme could interfere with this process. Alternatively, this enzyme also functions *in vitro* to release coenzyme A from palmitoyl-CoA; it is possible that lack of this activity may adversely affect fatty acid metabolism in neurons.

Your patient has NEURONAL CEROID LIPOFUSCINOSIS.

REFERENCES

Camp, L. A., Verkruyse, L. A., Afendis, S. J., Slaughter, C. A., and Hofmann, S. L. Molecular cloning and expression of palmitoyl-protein thioesterase. *J. Biol. Chem.* 269: 23212, 1994.

Vesa, J., Helisten, E., Verkruyse, L. A., Camp, L. A., Rapola, J., Santavuori, P., Hofmann, S. L., and Peltonen, L. Mutations in the palmitoyl protein thioesterase gene causing infantile neuronal ceroid lipofuscinosis. *Nature* 376: 584, 1995.

Answer 88

a. First, analyze the nature of the mutation:

Codon number:	242	243	244	245	246	247	248	249	250
Normal person:									
DNA:	AAG	ATC	ACG	CTG	TGC	ATC	TCC	GTG	CTG
RNA:	AAG	AUC	ACG	CUG	UGC	AUC	UCC	GUG	CUG
Protein:	Lys	Ilu	Thr	Leu	Cys	Ilu	Ser	Val	Leu
Your patient:									
DNA:	AAG	ATC	ACG	CTG	TGC	ATC	TTC	GTG	CTG
RNA:	AAG	AUC	ACG	CUG	UGC	AUC	UUC	GUG	CUG
Protein:	Lys	Ilu	Thr	Leu	Cys	Ilu	Phe	Val	Leu

The mutation replaces a serine at position 248 with a phenylalanine. This is clearly a position that is highly conserved. A large variety of acetylcholine receptors have either a serine at this position or a threonine, but no other residue. To replace the serine with a phenylalanine is likely to have a drastic effect on the function. The mutation is in a transmembrane α-helical portion of the receptor. There appear to be in a given organism a total of 10 different forms of the receptor protein. These function by complexing in groups of 5, arranging themselves such that five α-helices form a pentameric channel, which can become permeable to cations such as sodium and potassium. The pentameric channel consists of 5 α-helices such as the one that, in α4, contains serine 248. Even if these α-helices are from different types of subunit, their sequences are very similar, and as shown above, serine 248 and leucine 251 are highly conserved. Any given complex may consist of different combinations of subunits. It is not clear exactly which combinations occur in particular cases.

In the function of the nicotinic acetylcholine receptor, serine 248 and leucine 251 play critical roles. In the absence of acetyl-

NORMAL PERSON

Acetylcholine Bound to Receptor

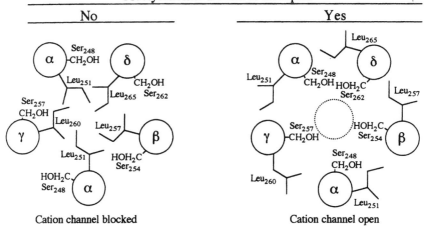

No	Yes
Cation channel blocked	Cation channel open

YOUR PATIENT

Acetylcholine Bound to Receptor

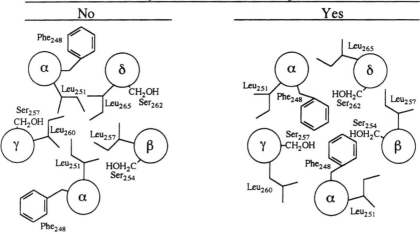

No	Yes
Cation channel blocked	Cation channel blocked

FIGURE A88-1. **Function of the acetylcholine receptor.** The transmembrane portion of the acetylcholine receptor consists of various helices, of which the five that form the cation channel are shown. These helices are from the α, β, γ, and δ subunits of the receptor, the α chains contributing two and the others one each. In a normal person (top), in the absence of acetylcholine, the helices are oriented such that hydrophobic leucine residues prevent cations from passing through the channel (top left); when acetylcholine binds to the receptor (top right), the helices rotate and the side chains of the polar serine residues form a channel permeable to cations. In your patient, however, ser248 in the α subunit is changed to phe248 (bottom). This does not affect the closure of the channel in the absence of acetylcholine (bottom left), but when acetylcholine binds to the receptor, the helices rotate so that the hydrophobic side chains of phe248 are blocking the cation channel (bottom right).

choline, the α-helical region containing these residues is oriented such that the side chains of leucine 251 and its equivalents in the other α-helices form a hydrophobic ring that prevents cations from passing through. When acetylcholine binds to the receptor, the α-helices move so that the leucine side chains are no longer blocking passage of cations and, instead, the polar side chains of serine 248 and its equivalents form a ring that facilitates passage of cations. Replacing serine 248 with a hydrophobic phenylalanine is likely to inhibit passage of cations through the channel.

b. It is not clear why the disease is confined to the frontal lobe and occurs only during sleep. A significant fact is that it is likely different nicotinic acetylcholine receptor molecules may differ from each other in their content of the α4 subunit, with some having only one and others having two. It is probable that the latter would have their function more seriously compromised by the mutation. It is possible, although not certain, that the frontal lobe may have a higher concentration of the α4 subunit than other parts of the brain.

During sleep, certain neuronal systems are active, some of which may not be active during the waking state. The converse is also true. Perhaps some of these neuronal interactions require nicotinic cholinergic receptors that happen to have a higher proportion of α4 subunits. If these subunits are defective, then one might expect that aberrant neurotransmission could occur, leading to a brief seizure. When the patient is awake, other neuronal interactions, perhaps involving fewer α4 subunits, could take over and suppress any aberrant activity.

Your patient has AUTOSOMAL DOMINANT NOCTURNAL FRONTAL LOBE EPILEPSY.

REFERENCES

Devillers-Thiéry, A., Galzi, J. L., Eiselé, J. L., Bertrand, S., Bertrand, D., and Changeux, J. P., Functional architecture of the nicotinic acetylcholine receptor: A prototype of ligand-gated ion chanels. *J. Membrane Biol.* 136: 97, 1993.

Goto, K. The on-off mechanisms of the nicotinic acetylcholine receptor ion channel are performed by thermodynamic forces. *J. Theor. Biol.* 170: 267, 1994.

Scheffer, I. E., Bhatia, K. P., Lopes-Cendes, I., Fish, D. R., Marsden, C. D.,

Andermann, E., Andermann, F., Desbiens, R., Keene, D., Cendes, F., Manson, J. I., Constantinou, J. E. C., McIntosh, A., and Berkovic, S. F. Autosomal dominant nocturnal frontal lobe epilepsy. A distinctive clinical disorder. *Brain* 118: 61, 1995.

Steinlein, O. K., Mulley, J. C., Propping, P., Wallace, R. H., Phillips, H. A., Sutherland, G. R., Scheffer, I. E., and Berkovic, S. F. A missense mutation in the neuronal nicotinic acetylcholine repector α4 subunit is associated with autosomal dominant nocturnal frontal lobe epilepsy. *Nat. Genet.* 11: 201, 1995.

Steriade, M., McCormick, D. A., and Sejnowski, T. J., Thalamocortical oscillations in the sleeping and aroused brain. *Science* 262: 679, 1993.

Unwin, N. Nicotinic acetylcholine receptor at 9 Å resolution. *J. Mol. Biol.* 229: 1101, 1993.

Answer 89

a. Preproendothelin-3 is the precursor of the peptide endothelin-3, which is one of a family of biologically active peptides, the others being endothelin-1 and endothelin-2 (Fig. A89-1). The function of endothelin-2 is not known, but endothelin-1 is one of the most potent known vasoconstrictors. In contrast, endothelin-3 appears to be involved in embryonic development, particularly that of neurons.

Begin by analyzing the mutation:

Codon number:	156	157	158	159	160
Normal person:					
DNA:	CAC	TTG	CGC	TGC	GCT
RNA:	CAC	UUG	CGC	UGC	GCU
Protein:	His	Leu	Arg	Cys	Ala
Your patient:					
DNA:	CAC	TTG	CGC	TTC	GCT
RNA:	CAC	UUG	CGC	UUC	GCU
Protein:	His	Leu	Arg	Phe	Ala

Your patient's preproendothelin-3 has a phenylalanine at position 159 instead of a cysteine. Position 159 is not part of the mature endothelin-3 peptide, so it may not be immediately apparent why a mutation at this position could be harmful. However, the positions of the cysteines provide a clue. Residues 97 to 117 of pre-

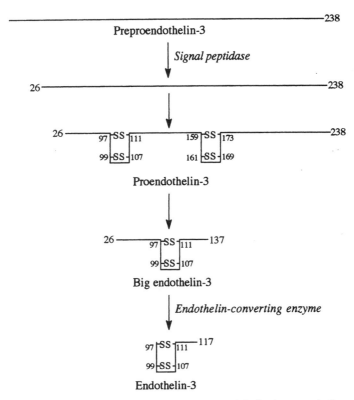

FIGURE A89-1. **Synthesis of endothelin-3.** The disulfide bridges are indicated. The disulfide loop involving residues 159 to 173 is hypothetical.

proendothelin-3 constitute the future biologically active endothelin-3. Cysteines 97, 99, 107, and 111 of preproendothelin-3 become cysteines 1, 3, 11, and 15 of the mature endothelin-3. The latter has disulfides joining cysteines 1 and 15 and cysteines 3 and 11. These disulfides are thought to be very important to the function of endothelin-3, because substituting cysteines with other residues greatly reduces the activity. Later in the sequence of preproendothelin-3 are residues 159 to 173 whose sequence is very similar to that of endothelin-3. In fact, in this endothelin-like sequence, the cysteines (at positions 159, 161, 169, and 173) are in precisely the same order as in endothelin-3. This raises the question of what the role of this region is. It could be the precursor to another endothelin-like peptide that has not yet been discovered. It could also be that the cysteines form disulfides and give this segment an appearance similar to that of the segment that will give rise to endothelin-3. It could conceivably play a role in recognizing the proteolytic enzyme whose action generates endothelin-3. The mutation in your patient removes one of these cysteines. It is possible that this inhibits the proteolytic processing and, hence, that at crucial stages of early development, your patient will not have the endothelin-3 levels she needs in order to have proper development of her neural crest. The neural crest gives rise to migrating cells including inner ear cells, parasympathetic enteric neurons, and melanocytes. If your patient lacks endothelin-3, then she will have poor innervation of the colon (constipation), deafness, and improper pigmentation.

b. Preproendothelin-3 is cleaved by signal peptidase to generate proendothelin-3, which is then cleaved to generate big endothelin-3, which is then cleaved by a metalloproteinase called endothelin-converting enzyme to generate endothelin-3. The latter enzyme is an unusual one because it cleaves between a tryptophan and an isoleucine.

c. There are two receptors for the endothelins. The endothelin-A receptor has 10 times as great an affinity for endothelin-1 than for endothelin-3; it is located on vascular smooth-muscle cells and largely mediates the action of endothelin-1 on blood pressure. The endothelin-B receptor is located mainly on endothelial cells and has an equal affinity for endothelin-1 and endothelin-3. It plays a critical role in the development of cells derived from neural crest precursors. Thus, even though both endothelins bind to the same receptors, they do not bind equally well to the two receptors, hence, their effects *in vivo* can be very different.

Your patient has SHAH-WAARDENBURG SYNDROME.

REFERENCES

Baynash, A. G., Hosoda, K., Giaid, A., Richardson, J. A., Emoto, N., Hammer, R. E., and Yanagisawa, M. Interaction of endothelin-3 with endothelin-B receptor is essential for development of epidermal melanocytes and enteric neurons. *Cell* 79: 1277, 1994.

Bloch, K. D., Eddy, R. L., Shows, T. B., and Quertermous, T. cDNA cloning and chromosomal assignment of the gene encoding endothelin 3. *J. Biol. Chem.* 264: 18156, 1989.

Edery, P., Attié, T., Amiel, J., Pelet, A., Eng, C., Hofstra, R. M. W., Martelli, H., Bidaud, C., Munnich, A., and Lyonnete, S. Mutation of the endothelin-3 gene in the Waardenburg-Hirschsprung disease (Shah-Waardenburg syndrome). *Nat. Genet.* 12: 442, 1996.

Hofstra, R. M. W., Osinga, J., Tan-Sindhunata, G., Wu, Y., Kamsteeg, E.-J., Stulp, R. P., van Ravenswaaij-Arts, C., Majoor-Krakauer, D., Angrist, M., Chakravarti, A., Meijers, C., and Buys, C. H. C. M. A homozygous mutation in the endothelin-3 gene associated with a combined Waardenburg type 2 and Hirschsprung phenotype (Shah-Waardenburg syndrome). *Nat. Genet.* 12: 445, 1996.

Inoue, A., Yanagisawa, M., Kimura, S., Kasuya, Y., Miyauchi, T., Goto, K., and Masaki, T. The human endothelin family: Three structurally and pharmacologically distinct isopeptides predicted by three separate genes. *Proc. Natl. Acad. Sci. USA* 86: 2963, 1989.

Levin, E. R. Endothelins. *N. Engl. J. Med.* 333: 356, 1995.

Sakurai, T., Yanagisawa, M., and Masaki, T. Molecular characterization of endothelin receptors. *Trends Pharm. Sci.* 13: 103, 1992.

Shiba, R., Sakurai, T., Yamada, G., Morimoto, H., Saito, A., Masaki, T., and Goto, K. Cloning and expression of rat preproendothelin-3 cDNA. *Biochem. Biophys. Res. Commun.* 186: 588, 1992.

Xu, D., Emoto, N., Giaid, A., Slaughter, C., Kaw, S., deWit, D., Yanagisawa, M. ECE-1: A membrane-bound metalloprotease that catalyzes the proteolytic activation of big endothelin-1. *Cell* 78: 473, 1994.

Yanagisawa, M., and Masaki, T. Molecular biology and biochemistry of the endothelins. *Trends Pharm. Sci.* 10: 374, 1989.

Zoghbi, H. Y., and Ballabio, A. Waardenburg syndrome. C. R. Scriver, A. L. Beaudet, W. S. Sly, and D. Valle (Eds.). *The Metabolic and Molecular Bases of Inherited Disease.* New York: McGraw-Hill, 1995, Vol. III, Chap. 154D, p. 4575.

CHAPTER 17

Cancer

Problem 90

Your patient has colon cancer. From a biopsy sample, you have discovered that he has an altered gene. In his noncancerous tissues, your patient has a normal gene. The alteration is shown here:

Codon number:	250	251	252	253	254
Normal gene:	AAC	TAC	TCA	GTG	AAG
Altered gene:	AAC	TAC	TAA	GTG	AAG

The overall sequence of the gene is similar to that of a protein from yeast called mutL.

Based on this information, how might the mutation lead to the disease?

Problem 91

Your patient has prostate cancer. In his tumor cells he has an alteration in a protein called Mxi1. The alteration is shown here:

Codon number: 138   139 140 141   142 143 144 145 146
Normal person: AGA TTT TTA AAG TGG CGA CTG GAA CAG
Your patient: AGA TTT TTA AGT GGC GAC TGG AAC AGC

You clone and express both your patient's abnormal Mxi1 and normal Mxi1. You also obtain other proteins called Max and c-Myc and mix them in different combinations with each other and with a piece of DNA containing the c-Myc binding site. You then do an electrophoretic mobility shift assay in which you look to see which of these combinations binds to the DNA. Here are the results (remember, every combination includes the DNA containing the c-Myc binding site):

Proteins Added				
Normal Mxi1	Your patient's Mxi1	c-Myc	Max	DNA Binding
Yes	No	No	No	No
No	Yes	No	No	No
No	No	Yes	No	No
No	No	No	Yes	No
No	No	Yes	Yes	Yes
Yes	No	No	Yes	Yes
No	Yes	No	Yes	No

a. What is the functional relationship between c-Myc, Max, and Mxi1?

b. What kind of mutation occurred in this protein and how might the mutation cause the tumor?

Problem 92

Your patient has a malignant lung carcinoma. The tumor cells have a gene that is expressed in elevated amounts compared to normal cells. The gene codes for a protein of 582 amino acids. The protein has many homologies to stromelysin and progelatinase A. It also has a region of unusual sequence (positions 539 to 562):

AAAVVLPVLLLLLVLAVGLAVFFF

When this protein is incubated with progelatinase A, the latter is cleaved into smaller pieces. Progelatinase A is generally expressed by the stromal cells surrounding the tumor rather than by the tumor cells themselves.

a. Put these facts together to account for why this protein is expressed in elevated levels in malignant tumors.

b. What might be the significance of the unusual sequence at positions 539 to 562?

Problem 93

Your patient with a malignant melanoma has asked you if you might be treating his cancer with a drug that targets telomerase. He saw telomerase mentioned on the television news and it aroused his hopes. You have to tell him that at the moment no such drug exists.

a. What is the mechanism of action of telomerase? Comment on its structure.

b. Why is it an attractive target for cancer chemotherapy?

Problem 94

Your patient has polyps in his colon. You do a biopsy and find that he has an altered gene. You are able to purify the altered gene product as well as the equivalent protein from a normal individual. You do the following experiments and obtain the indicated results:

1. You find that the normal protein binds strongly to β-catenin. The altered protein binds weakly to it.

2. You find that the normal protein strongly promotes tubulin polymerization *in vitro,* while the altered protein is unable to do this.

3. You do immunofluorescence using an antibody that recognizes either the normal or the altered protein. You find that cells containing the normal protein stain in a filamentous pattern, while cells containing the altered protein give a diffuse pattern. If you incubate the cells containing the normal protein with nocodazole, the filamentous staining pattern is replaced with a diffuse one.

a. What is the likely role of this protein?

b. Why does the mutation lead to the symptoms?

Problem 95

Many people in China and South Africa who have liver cancer have a somatic mutation at residue 249 in a protein called p53. The mutations are shown here:

    Codon number: 249
    Normal person: AGG
    Patient 1:   AGT
    Patient 2:   AGC

Many people with tumors have mutations in p53, at various positions in the sequence, but many people with liver cancer from these two parts of the world have one of the mutations shown above, and only at position 249.

a. Liver cancer is a rare disease. Why would a variety of unrelated people living in two different parts of the world get liver cancer and have their causative mutation in the same codon, particularly when mutations in other parts of the protein can cause other cancers? Think of two possible explanations. Hint: Aflatoxin is a common contaminant of food in the countries mentioned.

b. What is the mechanism of action of aflatoxin B_1?

c. How might the mutation lead to the disease?

Problem 96

In 1967, Vice President Hubert Humphrey checked into Bethesda Naval Hospital after observing blood in his urine. The diagnosis at the time was cystitis in his bladder. Two years later, he was diagnosed with bladder cancer. Gradually the cancer worsened until Humphrey died in 1978. In 1976, a biopsy was performed and the tissue frozen. Recently, the tissue was examined and an alteration was found in the gene for p53. The alteration is shown here:

Codon number:	226	227	228	229
Normal person:	GGC	TCT	GAC	TGT
Your patient:	GGC	TCA	GAC	TGT

How could the mutation lead to the tumor? Hint: Look up Figure 1 on page 260 in *Methods in Enzymology*, Vol. 183 (1990).

Problem 97

The argument has been made that if drugs such as taxol and taxotere could be modified so that they could cross the blood–brain barrier more readily, such modified drugs might be a promising treatment for Alzheimer's disease.

a. Knowing the target for taxol and taxotere, explain the rationale for this argument.

b. What might be a good argument against using these drugs for Alzheimer's disease?

Problem 98

Your patient has a fatty tumor. Further study reveals that he has chimeric RNA transcripts, consisting of the DNA binding domain of HMGI-C fused to transcriptional regulatory domains.

   a. What is the function of HMGI-C?

   b. How might this mutation lead to the disease?

Problem 99

Your patient is a 35-year-old woman with a sarcoma. Her mother and her brother also had sarcomas when they were in their 30s. You observe that there is a mutation in the gene for p53, a protein with five exons. The mutation is at the beginning of the fourth intron, where there is an AT instead of a GT. You prepare and sequence the cDNAs for her p53 and you find that she has two cDNAs. One lacks part of exon 4 and the other lacks all of exon 4.

a. How could the mutation lead to the production of two different mRNAs for p53?

b. How could this aberrant p53 cause the disease?

Answer 90

The mutation is analyzed as follows:

Codon number:	250	251	252	253	254
Normal person's DNA:	AAC	TAC	TCA	GTG	AAG
Normal person's RNA:	AAC	UAC	UCA	GUG	AAG
Normal person's protein:	Asn	Tyr	Ser	Val	Lys
Your patient's DNA:	AAC	TAC	TAA	GTG	AAG
Your patient's RNA:	AAC	UAC	UAA	GUG	AAG
Your patient's protein:	Asn	Tyr	STOP		

Your patient's protein has a termination codon at position 252 instead of a serine. Thus, whatever the function of the protein, in the tumor the protein is probably nonfunctional.

The homologous protein in yeast, mutL, is a DNA mismatch repair enzyme, which excises mismatched bases. This type of enzyme is useful for eliminating mutations. If your patient's enzyme has the same job, then you could imagine that without a "policeman" to find and delete mismatched DNA, other mutations could appear, some of which could lead to uncontrolled proliferation, or, in a word, a tumor. This particular protein is called hMLH1.

Your patient has NONPOLYPOSIS COLON CANCER.

REFERENCES

Papadopoulos, N., Nicolaides, N. C., Wei, Y.-F., Ruben, S. M., Carter, K. C., Rosen, C. A., Haseltine, W. A., Fleischmann, R. D., Fraser, C. M., Adams, M. D., Venter, J. C., Hamilton, S. R., Petersen, G. M., Watson, P., Lynch, H. T., Peltomäki, P., Mecklin, J.-P., de la Chapelle, A., Kinzler, K. W., and Vogelstein, B. Mutation of a *mutL* homolog in hereditary colon cancer. *Science* 263: 1625, 1994.

Answer 91

a. c-Myc is a transcription factor that binds to a region on DNA and stimulates the transcription of proteins involved in cellular proliferation. In order to bind to DNA, c-Myc has to dimerize with Max. Max also forms dimers with Mxi1. These dimers also bind to the c-Myc binding site on DNA. Unlike the c-Myc/Max complex, the Mxi1/Max complex inhibits transcription. Thus, the Mxi1/Max complex competes with the c-Myc/Max complex (Fig. A91-1).

b. The mutation is analyzed as follows:

Codon number:	138	139	140	141	142	143	144	145	146
Normal person's DNA:	AGA	TTT	TTA	AAG	TGG	CGA	CTG	GAA	CAG
Normal person's RNA:	AGA	UUU	UUA	AAG	UGG	CGA	CUG	GAA	CAG
Normal person's protein:	Arg	Phe	Leu	Lys	Trp	Arg	Leu	Glu	Gln
Your patient's DNA:	AGA	TTT	TTA	AGT	GGC	GAC	TGG	AAC	AGC
Your patient's RNA:	AGA	UUU	UUA	AGU	GGC	GAC	UGG	AAC	AGC
Your patient's protein:	Arg	Phe	Leu	Ser	Gly	Asp	Trp	Asn	Ser

Your patient's Mxi1 has a deletion of an A in codons 140 or 141. This results in a frame shift mutation. Frame shift mutations can be catastrophic, since the entire sequence of the protein after the site of the deletion could change. Presumably, therefore, these tumor cells have a nonfunctional Mxi1 protein. Since Mxi1 is part of the system by which activity of c-Myc is controlled, loss of Mxi1 means that c-Myc activity will increase greatly, resulting in expression of factors causing cell proliferation and thus resulting in a tumor (Fig. A91-2).

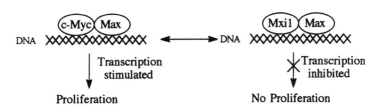

FIGURE A91-1. **Roles of c-Myc, Max, and Mxi1 in transcription.** In the presence of Max, transcription by c-Myc is stimulated; this leads to production of proteins that cause proliferation. In contrast, Mxi1 inhibits transcription when it complexes with Max. Mxi1, and c-Myc bind to the same site on DNA. Thus, the equilibrium between Max binding to c-Myc and Max binding to Mxi1 acts to regulate the level of proliferation.

NORMAL PERSON

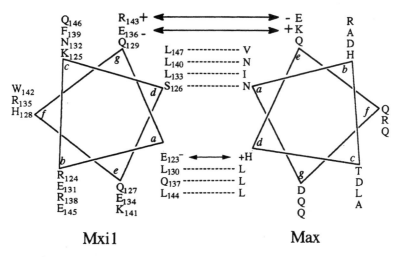

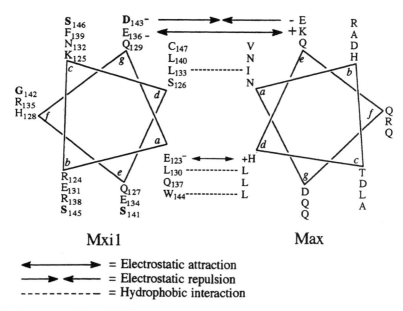

FIGURE A91-2. Effect of the mutation in Mxi1 on its binding to Max. The diagram gives end-on views of the α-helices in Mxi1 and Max, showing the region where the two proteins bind to each other. *Top*: In an α-helix, every residue is directly below the residue seven positions away from it in the amino acid sequence. The seven positions are assigned the letters *a,, b, c, d, e, f,* and *g.* As you can see in the diagram, in a normal person there are electrostatic interactions between two

REFERENCES

Eagle, L. R., Yin, X., Brothman, A. R., Williams, B. J., Atkin, N. B., and Prochownik, E. V. Mutation of the *MXI1* gene in prostate cancer. *Nat. Genet.* 9: 249, 1995.

Zervos, A., Gyuris, J., and Brent, R. Mxi1, a protein that specifically interacts with Max to bind Myc-Max recognition sites. *Cell* 72: 223, 1993.

Answer 92

a. The protein is evidently a proteolytic enzyme. In fact, it is a matrix metalloproteinase requiring zinc for its activity. It is produced by the tumor cells and cleaves the zymogen progelatinase A secreted by the stromal cells. The cleaved progelatinase A now becomes the active enzyme gelatinase A, which cleaves collagen IV, the major component of the basement membranes. As the basement membranes disappear, the tumor is able to grow and spread into new tissues; hence it is malignant. The fact that the gelatinase A becomes activated at the edge of the tumor is consistent with this hypothesis.

b. The region comprising positions 539 to 562 is a highly hydrophobic segment of 24 residues, about the right size to be a transmembrane domain. This metalloproteinase, therefore, is likely to be anchored to the membrane of the tumor cell. As the tumor grows, the metalloproteinase activates the progelatinase A of

---

residues in position *g* of Mxi1 and two in position *e* of Max and between one residue in position *a* of Mxi1 and position *d* of Max. Similarly, there are hydrophobic interactions between side chains in positions *a* and *d* of Mxi1 and positions *d* and *a* of Max. These interactions are what cause Mxi1 and Max to bind to each other. *Bottom*: The frame shift mutation that occurs in your patient is very deleterious to this arrangement. First, conversion of the positively charged arg143, which forms an electrostatic bond with a glutamate residue in Max, to a negatively charged asp143 changes electrostatic attraction into electrostatic repulsion. Second, changing the hydrophobic leu147 into the polar cys147 eliminates one of the hydrophobic interactions between Mxi1 and Max. Finally, conversion of the bulky trp142 to the tiny gly142 could have even more deleterious consequences: Since glycine destabilizes α-helices, it is possible that this mutation may disrupt this α-helix and thereby prevent Mxi1 binding to Max altogether.

the stromal cells with which the tumor comes into contact. If the hydrophobic domain were missing, and the metalloproteinase free in the extracellular matrix, its progelatinase A activation would be more randomly located and of little use to the tumor cell.

REFERENCES

Sato, H., Takino, T., Okada, Y., Cao, J., Shinagawa, A., Yamamoto, E., and Seiki, M. A matrix metalloproteinase expressed on the surface of invasive tumour cells. *Nature* 370: 61, 1994.

Answer 93

a. Telomerase (Fig. A93-1) is an enzyme adapted to literally take care of a "loose end" in DNA replication. When DNA replicates, the DNA polymerase III synthesizes DNA in the $5' \rightarrow 3'$ direction. For one strand (the leading strand), DNA polymerization is straightforward: As the DNA unwinds, an RNA polymerase called primase synthesizes a short segment of RNA (8 to 12 bases) complementary to the parent DNA strand. Then the DNA polymerase III moves directly to copy the newly exposed single-stranded DNA. For the lagging strand, however, the $5' \rightarrow 3'$ direction is opposite to that of the unwinding. For this strand, therefore, the new DNA needs to be synthesized in small segments (called Okazaki fragments). In this more complex process, primase synthesizes a segment of RNA complementary to the DNA. Then DNA polymerase III moves in to extend that RNA primer as DNA. Then the $5' \rightarrow 3'$ exonuclease activity of DNA polymerase I removes the RNA primer, after which DNA polymerase I fills the gap until a DNA ligase ties the pieces together. Although cumbersome, this procedure does the job very effectively, except at the end of the strand. Removal of the RNA primer at this position leaves a gap that DNA polymerase cannot fill since it needs the primer. Thus, the end of the replication process will leave a short segment of single-stranded DNA at the end of the lagging strand. This loose end would soon be degraded by the action of nucleases in the cell. One can imagine that it would be unfortunate if every

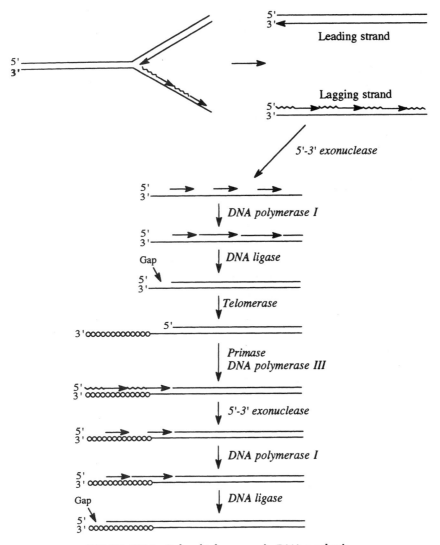

FIGURE A93-1. **Role of telomerase in DNA synthesis.**

cycle of replication were followed by loss of DNA. Eventually, important genes would start to disappear.

This is where *telomerase* comes in. This enzyme has the unusual activity of adding some nucleotides to the 3' ends of the DNA prior to replication. Thus, when the ends are lost during replication, no harm is done because only the telomeric DNA, added by the telomerase activity, disappears. The essential DNA remains intact. The specifics of the process appear to be the following. First, telomerase adds several hundred nucleotides to the 3' end of the DNA. Then conventional DNA replication takes place, with the action of a primase followed by an as yet uncharacterized DNA polymerase activity that replicates the telomeric DNA. As expected, a small segment of the telomeric DNA is lost in the process.

The telomerase enzyme is an unusual one. It contains a small RNA template. The telomeric DNA it synthesizes consists of numerous copies complementary to this template. In humans, the RNA template has the sequence CUAACCCUAAC. This template codes for the human telomere sequence (TTAGGG)$_n$.

b. The existence of telomerase has several important implications. For one, it is tempting to explain aging as due in part to loss of telomerase activity. If, after each replication, a little DNA is lost, eventually the functional DNA of a cell will begin to disappear and the cell will become less healthy until it ultimately dies. Conversely, telomerase activity is often elevated in immortalized cells such as tumors. The telomerase activity allows the cells to replicate indefinitely. It is attractive to speculate that inhibition of telomerase will cause cancer cells to become like normal cells, namely, to become mortal and eventually die. For this reason, there is presently a great deal of research dedicated to developing a drug that inhibits telomerase.

REFERENCES

Greider, C. W. and Blackburn, E. H. Telomeres, telomerase and cancer. *Sci. Am.* 274: 92, 1996.

Holliday, R. Endless quest. *BioEssays* 18: 3

Kim, N. W., Piatyszek, M. A., Prowse, K. R., Harley, C. B., West, M. D., Ho, P. L. C., Coviello, G. M., Wright, W. E., Weinrich, S. L., and Shay, J. W. Specific association of human telomerase activity with immortal cells and cancer. *Science* 266: 2011, 1994.

Sharma, H. W., Maltese, J.-Y., Zhu, X., Kaiser, H. E., and Narayanan, R. Telomeres, telomerase and cancer: is the magic bullet real? *Anticancer Res.* 16: 511, 1996.

Zakian, V. A. Telomeres: Beginning to understand the end. *Science* 270: 1601, 1995.

Answer 94

a. The protein is called APC. The normal protein is able to bind to both tubulin and β-catenin. The fact that APC gives filamentous staining, which is turned diffuse by the microtubule-disrupting agent nocodazole, suggests that APC is associated with microtubules. This is confirmed by the fact that it enhances tubulin polymerization *in vitro*. APC also binds to β-catenin, a protein that binds to an adhesion molecule called E-cadherin. In a sense, APC helps to connect the adhesion network to the cytoskeleton.

b. The altered APC is unable to bind to microtubules and it binds weakly to β-catenin. This suggests that it is unable to organize the adhesion of one cell to another. In other words, cell adhesion is weakened. This would imply that cells would grow and divide more aggressively, resulting in these benign growths.

Your patient has ADENOMATOUS POLYPOSIS COLI.

REFERENCES

Munemitsu, S., Souza, B., Müller, O., Albert, I., Rubinfeld, B., and Polakis, P. The APC gene product associates with microtubules *in vivo* and promotes their assembly *in vitro*. *Cancer Res.* 54: 3676, 1994.

Rubinfeld, B., Souza, B., Albert, I., Müller, O., Chamberlain, S. H., Masiarz, F. R., Munemitsu, S., and Polakis, P. Association of the *APC* gene product with β-catenin. *Science* 262: 1731, 1993.

Smith, K. J., Levy, D. B., Maupin, P., Pollard, T. D., Vogelstein, B., and Kinzler, K. W. Wild-type but not mutant APC associates with the microtubule cytoskeleton. *Cancer Res.* 54: 3672, 1994.

Su, L.-K., Vogelstein, B., and Kinzler, K. W. Association of the APC tumor suppressor protein with catenins. *Science* 262: 1734, 1993.

Answer 95

a. 1. A common causative agent, such as aflatoxin B_1, might have an affinity for one particular sequence in the DNA. Presumably, toxins such as this would be accumulated in the liver,

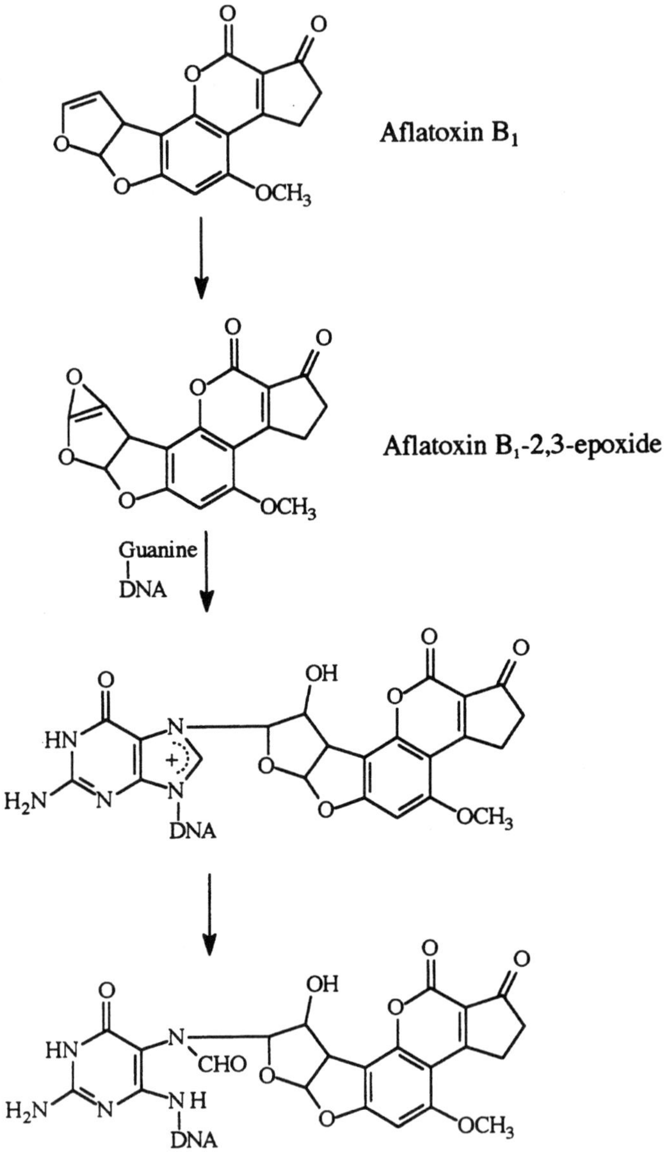

FIGURE A95-1. **Mechanism of action of aflatoxin B₁.** Aflatoxin B₁ is first metabolized to the epoxide, which reacts with guanine residues to generate an abnormal structure, which causes incorrect base pairing of DNA and thus leads to mutations.

which would therefore be vulnerable to this mutation. It would be of interest to see if patients with liver cancer in America or Europe, where aflatoxin B_1 is not a common contaminant, also have mutations at codon 249 in p53.

2. Cells containing p53 mutated at position 249 might replicate faster in the liver environment than cells containing either normal p53 or another mutant of p53.

b. Aflatoxin B_1 is a potent carcinogen that forms deoxyguanosine adducts and causes $G \rightarrow T$ transversions. It is metabolized to aflatoxin B_1-2,3-epoxide, the active form (Fig. A95-1). It is a common contaminant of food such as groundnuts, which form a staple among the poorer people in places such as Mozambique and Transkei (in southern Africa). It is also a common contaminant in corn in China.

c. Arginine 249 in p53 is next to arginine 248, which bonds to the DNA in the minor groove. The δ carbon of arginine 249 is in a Van der Waals contact with the side chain of histidine 162. The guanidinium group of arginine 249 is stacked against the side chain of tyrosine 163. The arginine may play a role in stabilizing the structure of that portion of p53, which interacts with DNA. Replacing the arginine with a much smaller serine would cause these interactions to be lost and the structure of the region binding the DNA would be destabilized. p53 would thus be inhibited from playing its role as a tumor suppressor.

REFERENCES

Autrup, H., Harris, C. C., Wu, S.-M., Bao, L. Y., Pei, X.-F., Lu, S., Sun, T.-T., and Hsia, C.-C. Activation of chemical carcinogens by cultured human fetal liver, esophagus and stomach. *Chem. Biol. Interact.* 50: 15, 1984.

Bressac, B., Kew, M., Wands, J., and Ozturk, M. Selective G to T mutations of p53 gene in hepatocellular carcinoma from southern Africa. *Nature* 350: 429, 1991.

Cho, Y., Gorina, S., Jeffrey, P. D., and Pavletich, N. P. Crystal structure of a p53 tumor suppressor-DNA complex: Understanding tumorigenic mutations. *Science* 265: 346, 1994.

Hsu, I. C., Metcalf, R. A., Sun, T., Welsh, J. A., Wang, N. J., and Harris, C. C. Mutational hotspot in the p53 gene in human hepatocellular carcinomas. *Nature* 350: 427, 1991.

Sambamurti, K., Callahan, J., Luo, X., Perkins, C. P., Jacobsen, J. S., and Humayun, M. Z. Mechanisms of mutagenesis by a bulky DNA lesion at the guanine N7 position. *Genetics* 120: 863, 1988.

Van Rensburg, S. J., Cook-Mozaffari, P., Van Schalkwyk, D. J., Van Der Watt, J. J., Vincent, T. J., and Purchase, I. F. Hepatocellular carcinoma and dietary aflatoxin in Mozambique and Transkei. *Br. J. Cancer* 51: 713, 1985.

Yeh, F.-S., Yu, M. C., Mo, C.-C., Luo, S. Tong, M. J., and Henderson, B. E. Hepatitis B virus, aflatoxins, and hepatocellular carcinoma in southern Guangxi, China. *Cancer Res.* 49: 2506, 1989.

Answer 96

The site of the mutation is in exon 7 (residues 225 to 260). The mutation is analyzed as follows:

Codon number:	226	227	228	229
Normal person's DNA:	GGC	TCT	GAC	TGT
Normal person's RNA:	GGC	UCU	GAC	UGU
Normal person's protein:	Gly	Ser	Asp	Cys
Your patient's DNA:	GGC	TCA	GAC	TGT
Your patient's RNA:	GGC	UCA	GAC	UGU
Your patient's protein:	Gly	Ser	Asp	Cys

The change from T to A clearly does not alter the meaning of the codon, so we have to look elsewhere. The figure in *Methods in Enzymology* (Vol. 183, p. 260) suggests that the altered sequence has a potential 3' splice site:

GGCTC**AG**ACTGT

The splice site is underlined. Such sites, which are located in exons, are called "cryptic" splice sites. Conceivably, the creation of this splice site would allow an alternative splicing in which exon 6 (residues 187 to 224) is connected to codon 228 in exon 7. Not only do we lose codons 225 to 227, but the splicing will be shifted by one nucleotide, resulting in a frame shift mutation. If you follow the sequence, this is what will result:

Codon number:

228	229	230	231	232	233	234	235	236	237	238	239	240	241	242	243	244	245	246

Normal:

DNA:
GAC TGT ACC ACC ATC CAC TAC AAC TAC ATG TGT AAC AGT TCC TGC ATG GGC GGC ATG

RNA:
GAC UGU ACC ACC AUC CAC UAC AAC UAC AUG UGU AAC AGU UCC UGC AUG GGC GGC AUG

Protein:
Asp Cys Thr Thr Ile His Tyr Asn Tyr Met Cys Asn Ser Ser Cys Met Gly Gly Met

Mutant::

DNA:
ACT GTA CCA CCA TCC ACT ACA ACT ACA TGT GTA ACA GTT CCT GCA TGG GCG GCA TGA

RNA:
ACU GUA CCA CCA UCC ACU ACA ACU ACA UGU GUA ACA GUU CCU GCA UGG GCG GCA UGA

Protein:
Thr Val Pro Pro Ser Thr Thr Thr Thr Cys Val Thr Val Pro Ala Trp Ala Ala STOP

Not only do we have a stretch of a completely different sequence due to the frame shift, but at position 246, we introduce a termination codon. In other words, it is very likely that the mutated p53 will have no activity. Even if Vice President Humphrey had a normal p53 in these cells, the low level of active p53 may have permitted proliferation leading eventually to a tumor.

It is interesting to speculate what would have happened had present tools in molecular biology been available in 1967. Perhaps knowing he had cancer, Humphrey would not have run for president in 1968, or, conversely, the cancer could have been caught early and treated and Humphrey, remaining more vigorous longer, may have exerted even more of an influence on American politics.

REFERENCES

Culliton, B. J. Hubert Humphrey's bladder cancer. *Nature* 369: 13, 1994.

Hruban, R. H., van der Riet, P., Erozan, Y. S., and Sidransky, D. Molecular biology and the early detection of carcinoma of the bladder—the case of Hubert H. Humphrey. *N. Engl. J. Med.* 330: 1276, 1994.

Lamb, P. and Crawford, L. Characterization of the human p53 gene. *Mol. Cell. Biol.* 6: 1379, 1986.

Senapathy, P., Shapiro, M. B., and Harris, N. L. Splice junctions, branch point sites, and exons: Sequence statistics, identification, and applications to genome project. *Methods Enzymol.* 183: 252, 1990.

Answer 97

a. Taxol and taxotere target microtubules. They enhance microtubule assembly and inhibit microtubule disassembly. In fact, both drugs are very useful anticancer agents because they inhibit mitosis and cell proliferation. Microtubule assembly *in vitro*, and perhaps *in vivo* as well, is greatly enhanced by microtubule-associated proteins such as tau. Tau is subject to phosphorylation. For reasons that are not yet clear, tau is hyperphosphorylated in Alzheimer's disease. Hyperphosphorylated tau is less able to interact with tubulin and hence unable to enhance microtubule assembly. Presumably, due to the important role that neuronal microtubules have to play in axonal transport, the impaired microtubule assembly may be in part responsible for the decay of mental function that is part of Alzheimer's. A drug that promotes microtubule assembly in the absence of tau could, in theory, compensate for the decreased amount of functional tau.

b. A possible counterargument is that taxol operates *in vivo* by freezing microtubule dynamics rather than by enhancing microtubule assembly. In fact, taxol's effects on dynamics are not so different from those of colchicine, an inhibitor of microtubule assembly. The effect on dynamics requires much lower concentrations of taxol than does the enhancement of assembly. Thus, a potential major problem with using a taxol-like drug as a treatment for Alzheimer's disease, is that for the treatment to work, freezing dynamics alone may not be sufficient; one would have to enhance microtubule assembly. For this, one would need very high concentrations of the drug, much higher than those that are needed for freezing the dynamics of microtubules. It is hard to imagine that these concentrations would not simultaneously be very deleterious for mitotic cells, particularly those of the bone marrow and epithelia.

Another potential counterargument is that freezing microtubule dynamics, which would surely happen, since it requires lower concentrations of the drug, may itself interfere with microtubule function in the neuron and also be deleterious.

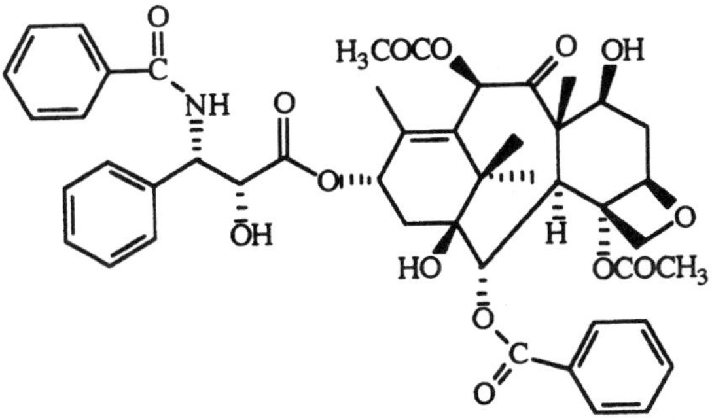

Taxol (Paclitaxel)

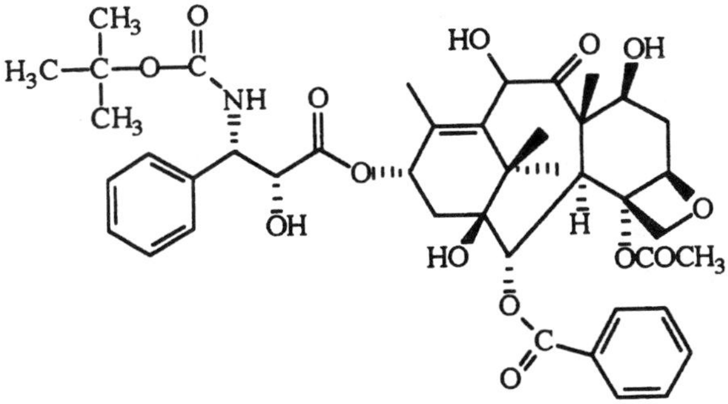

Taxotere (Docetaxel)

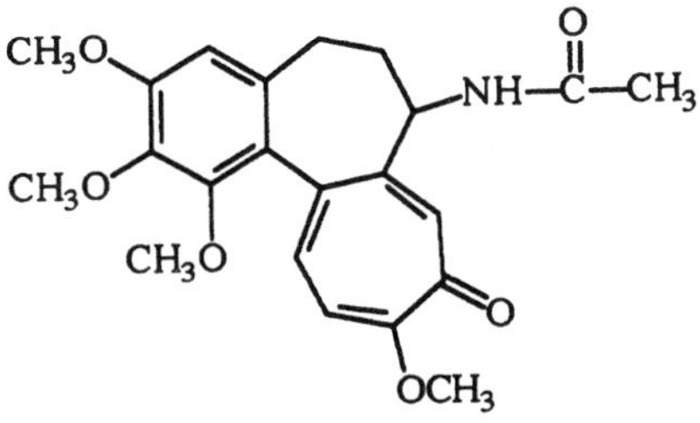

Colchicine

FIGURE A97-1. **Structures of taxol, taxotere, and colchicine.**

REFERENCES

Derry, B., Wilson, L., and Jordan, M. A. Substoichiometric binding of taxol suppresses microtubule dynamics. *Biochemistry* 34: 2203, 1995.

Jordan, M. A., Toso, R. J., Thrower, D. T., and Wilson, L. Mechanism of mitotic block and inhibition of cell proliferation by taxol at low concentrations. *Proc. Natl. Acad. Sci. USA* 90: 9552, 1993.

Lee, V. M.-Y., Daughenbaugh, R., and Trojanowski, J. Q. Microtubule stabilizing drugs for the treatment of Alzheimer's disease. *Neurobiol. Aging* 15, Suppl. 2: S87, 1994.

Panda, D., Daijo, J. E., Jordan, M. A., and Wilson, L. Kinetic stabilization of microtubule dynamics at steady state *in vitro* by substoichiometric concentrations of tubulin-colchicine complex. *Biochemistry* 34: 9921, 1995.

Answer 98

a. HMGCI-C is called an architectural transcription factor. Its function is to rearrange the structure of the DNA in such a way as to facilitate the binding of specific transcription factors.

b. Inappropriate activation of HMGI-C could lead to increased transcription of genes, stimulating in turn proliferation of the cells.

REFERENCES

Ashar, H. R., Schoenberg Fejzo, M., Tkachenko, A., Zhou, X., Fletcher, J. A., Weremowicz, S., Morton, C. C., and Chada, K. Disruption of the architectural factor HMGI-C: DNA binding AT hook motifs fused in lipomas to distinct transcriptional regulatory domains. *Cell* 82: 57, 1995.

Wolffe, A. P. Architectural transcription factors. *Science* 264: 1100, 1994.

Answer 99

a. The mutation at the beginning of the intron means that the splicing system will no longer recognize that particular splice site. Rather, it will splice the 3' end of exon 3 to the 5' end of exon 5, thereby leaving out all of exon 4. However, there is likely to be another GT in exon 4. Thus, the splicing system will recognize this as another ("cryptic") splice site and splice this to the 5' end of exon

NORMAL PERSON

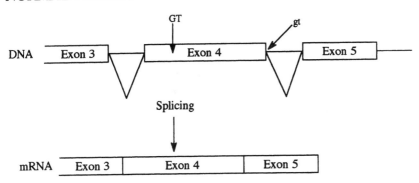

YOUR PATIENT

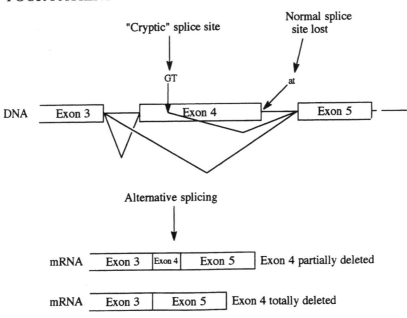

FIGURE A99-1. **Alternative splicing of mRNA in the Li–Fraumeni syndrome.** In a normal person (top), splicing occurs between exons 3, 4, and 5. In your patient (bottom), the "gt" splice site at the end of exon 4 has changed to an "at." This means that some of the splicing will occur between exon 3 and exon 5, deleting all of exon 4. However, there is a GT in exon 4; normally this is not involved in splicing. In the absence of the normal splice site, however, this GT becomes a cryptic splice site, resulting in splicing between this site in exon 4 and the beginning of exon 5. The result is a mRNA lacking some, but not all, of exon 4.

5. The result will be a mRNA lacking part, but not all, of exon 4 (Fig. A99-1).

b. Lacking all or part of exon 4, the function of p53 will be compromised. The result will be that p53 will not be able to inhibit proliferation and that will lead to a tumor.

Your patient has LI–FRAUMENI SYNDROME.

REFERENCES

Frebourg, T., Barbier, N., Yan, Y., Garber, J. E., Dreyfus, M., Fraumeni, J., Li, F. P., and Friend, S. H. Germ-line p53 mutations in 15 families with Li-Fraumeni syndrome. *Am. J. Hum. Genet.* 56: 608, 1995.

CHAPTER 18

Aging

Problem 100

In a recent study with the fruit fly *Drosophila,* researchers observed that transgenic flies overexpressing superoxide dismutase and catalase lived about 30% longer than normal flies. In another study, when *tert*-butyl-α-phenylnitrone was injected into senile gerbils, their mental acuity improved greatly. Put these findings together into a theory of aging. Speculate on how cellular proteins might be affected. What altered amino acids might you expect?

Answer 100

Superoxide dismutase and catalase destroy free radicals and other toxic by-products of oxidation. If not eliminated, free radicals react with proteins and other macromolecules and alter their functional behavior. Thus, the accumulation of free radicals is likely to oxidize proteins. This could gradually lead to loss of function and to cell death. A mark of this damage to proteins is the appearance of certain oxidized or otherwise altered amino acids. Some of these modified amino acids are given below (Fig. A100-1):

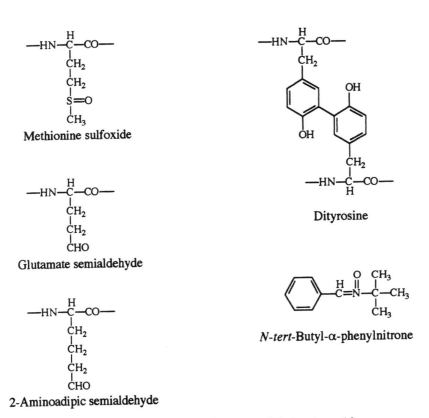

FIGURE A100-1. **Structures of some modified amino acids.**

Modified Residue	Product Formed
Proline	Glutamic semialdehyde, glutamate, 4-hydroxyproline
Arginine	Glutamic semialdehyde
Lysine	2-Aminoadipic semialdehyde
Histidine	Asparagine
Methionine	Methionine sulfoxide
Tyrosine	Dityrosine cross-links
Cysteine	Disulfides, lysinoalanine (Fig. 100-3)
Aspartate, asparagine	Isoaspartate (Fig. 100-2)
Asparagine	Aspartate

Which proteins are most susceptible to this type of damage? Obviously, proteins that turn over very slowly. This is probably the case with some of the structural proteins of neurons, which are cells that do not renew themselves. Likely candidates would be the neurofilament proteins and tubulin, the structural subunit of

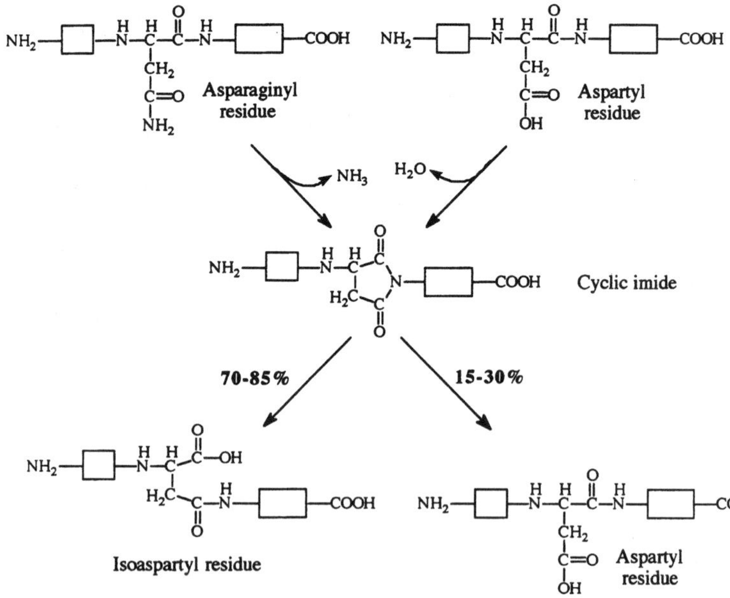

FIGURE A100-2. **Formation of isoaspartyl residues in proteins.** The diagram also shows how an asparagine residue can become an aspartate residue.

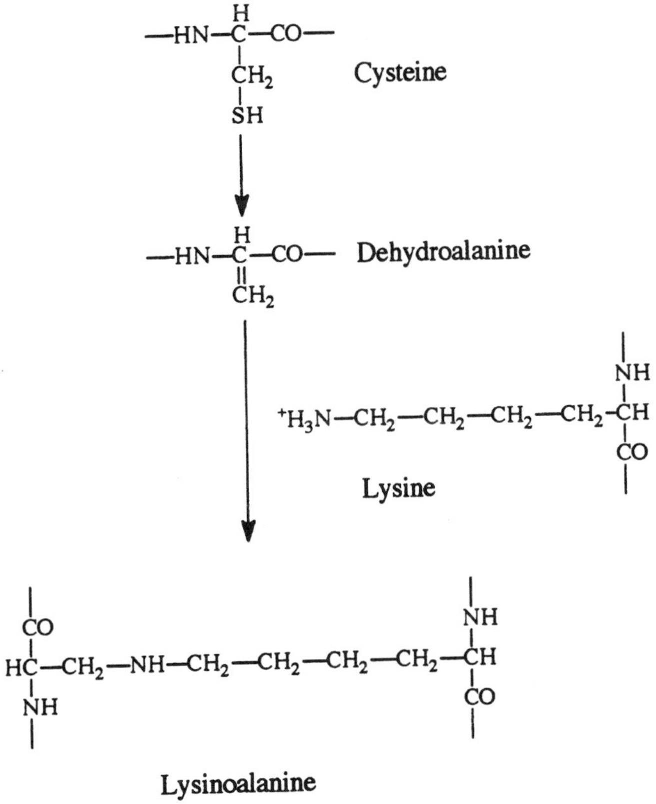

FIGURE A100-3. **Formation of lysinoalanine crosslinks in proteins.**

microtubules. Some of these modifications have been seen in tubulin purified from mammalian cerebra.

The compound *tert*-butyl-α-phenylnitrone also reacts with free radicals, hence, it would have a protective effect, as is true for the overexpression of superoxide dismutase and catalase. The fact that it seems to reverse senility in gerbils is particularly significant in that it points to the role of free radicals in the aging of neurons.

REFERENCES

Aeschbach, R., Amado, R., and Neukom, H. Formation of dityrosine cross-links in proteins by oxidation of tyrosine residues. *Biochim. Biophys. Acta* 439: 292, 1976.

Correia, J. J., Lipscomb, L. D., and Lobert, S. Nondisulfide crosslinking and chemical cleavage of tubulin subunits: pH and temperature dependence. *Arch. Biochem. Biophys.* 300: 105, 1993.

Najbauer, J., Orpiszewski, J., and Aswad, D. W. Molecular aging of tubulin: Accumulation of isoaspartyl sites in vitro and in vivo. *Biochemistry* 35: 5183, 1996.

Orr, W. C., and Sohal, R. S. Extension of life-span by overexpression of superoxide dismutase and catalase in *Drosophila melanogaster*. *Science* 263: 1128, 1994.

Stadtman, E. R. Protein oxidation and aging. *Science* 257: 1220, 1992.

Whitaker, J. R., and Feeney, R. E. Chemical and physical modification of proteins by the hydroxide ion. *Crit. Rev. Food Sci. Nutr.* 19: 173, 1983.

Index